MRCPsych PART I:
PASSING THE OSCE

MRCPsych PART I:
PASSING THE OSCE

Justin Sauer MBBS BSc MRCPsych
Specialist Registrar, Maudsley Hospital, London, UK

Colin O'Gara MB Bch BMedSci MRCPsych
Clinical Research Fellow, National Addiction Centre, Institute of
Psychiatry, London, UK

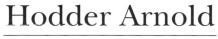

Hodder Arnold

A MEMBER OF THE HODDER HEADLINE GROUP

First published in Great Britain in 2005 by
Hodder Education, a member of the Hodder Headline Group,
338 Euston Road, London NW1 3BH

http://www.hoddereducation.co.uk

Distributed in the United States of America by
Oxford University Press Inc.,
198 Madison Avenue, New York, NY 10016
Oxford is a registered trademark of Oxford University Press

Whilst the advice and information in this book are believed to be true and
accurate at the date of going to press, neither the authors nor the publisher
can accept any legal responsibility or liability for any errors or omissions
that may be made. In particular, (but without limiting the generality of the
preceding disclaimer) every effort has been made to check drug dosages;
however, it is still possible that errors have been missed. Furthermore,
dosage schedules are constantly being revised and new side effects
recognised. For these reasons the reader is strongly urged to consult the
drug companies' printed instructions before administering any of the drugs
recommended in this book.

British Library Cataloguing in Publication Data
A catalogue record for this book is available from the British Library

Library of Congress Cataloging-in-Publication Data
A catalog record for this book is available from the Library of Congress

ISBN-10: 0 340 90472 0
ISBN-13: 978 0 340 90472 5

1 2 3 4 5 6 7 8 9 10

Commissioning Editor: Clare Christian
Project Editor: Clare Patterson
Production Controller: Jane Lawrence
Cover Design: Nichola Smith
Indexer: Laurence Errington

Typeset in 9.5 on 12pt Rotis Serif by Phoenix Photosetting Chatham, Kent
Printed and bound in Great Britain by CPI Bath

What do you think about this book? Or any other Hodder Arnold title?
Please visit our website at www.hoddereducation.co.uk

Dedicated to our families

CONTENTS

FOREWORD

For many of us for whom sitting the Membership is a distant memory, the recently introduced OSCE component of the Part I MRCPsych is rather baffling. Moving around a dozen (or more) stations in one and a half hours and making swift judgements about various clinical scenarios is very different to the clinical examination that the OSCE replaced.

However, the OSCE provides a much fairer and arguably more reliable examination method, since each candidate is asked the same questions in the same way and the use of actors ensures that mental state 'findings' are the same for everyone. Also, a much larger set of clinical situations can be examined than was possible in the previous single case clinical assessment.

For the candidate, a very specific set of skills have to be acquired. Careful attention to one's personal manner with 'patients' and their 'carers' under time constraints, thinking quickly and coherently about very different clinical scenarios each 7 minutes and being able to perform physical examinations correctly and competently are just some of the essential requirements.

This book provides excellent advice for those who have to acquire this expertise. Drs Justin Sauer and Colin O'Gara have written a comprehensive account of the logistics of the exam and give encouraging practical advice about pre-examination preparation and practise. (I particularly like the advice to practise interviewing skills with a television or radio playing to get used to the noise of other candidates at adjacent stations). Their worked case examples cover virtually every clinical scenario that the candidate is likely to meet. Most of all their writing style, while concise, is friendly and highly reassuring. I'm rather glad that I don't have to take an OSCE, but if I did, this is the first book I'd take off the shelf to help reduce my pre-exam nerves and prepare comprehensively.

Anne Farmer
Professor of Psychiatric Nosology
MRC SGDP Centre
Institute of Psychiatry
London, UK

PREFACE

The Objective Structured Clinical Examination (OSCE) is now an established component of the MRCPsych Part I, having been introduced by the Royal College of Psychiatrists in April 2003. Unfortunately, no examination method is liked by all candidates, and not everyone will be pleased with the change in format. However, the OSCE does have certain advantages, in particular elimination of the 'luck-of-the-draw' factor associated with examiner and patient selection in the Individual Patient Assessment (previously Part I). Now, all candidates are assessed at the same stations, by the same examiners, on the same patients (actors). There is an argument that this is fairer.

We have been preparing Part I candidates for the OSCE since late 2002 and continue to run courses twice a year. In this book, we plan to expose you to a wide range of OSCE experiences covering the majority of past questions and additional examples we believe are likely to come up.

A total of 96 individual stations have been set out in eight complete OSCEs. Practise them as mock examinations or individually – just make sure you practise.

Good luck!

Justin Sauer and Colin O'Gara

ACKNOWLEDGEMENTS

I am grateful to those who have had a positive and inspiring influence on me and also to all the OSCE candidates without whom this book would not have been possible.

Justin Sauer

I would like to thank Dr Michael Kelleher at the Institute of Psychiatry for his astute input over the past years.

Colin O'Gara

Thank you to our publishing colleagues at Hodder, who have been keen and encouraging throughout, in particular Clare Patterson, whose input has been invaluable.

With thanks to Dr David Gray and Dr Andrew Houghton for permission to use the ECG which appears in exam 8, and to Dr Paul Jenkins for permission to use the chest X-ray in exam 5. The artwork on pages 178 and 211 was drawn by Peter Richardson.

ABBREVIATIONS

A&E	Accident and Emergency
AN	anorexia nervosa
ANA	antinuclear antibody
A-V	arterio-venous
BDD	body dysmorphic disorder
BLS	basic life support
BMI	body mass index
BN	bulimia nervosa
BPAD	bipolar affective disorder
CBT	cognitive-behavioural therapy
CFS	chronic fatigue syndrome
CJD	Creutzfeldt–Jakob disease
CMHT	community mental health team
CN	cranial nerve
CNS	central nervous system
CPK	creatinine phosphokinase
CPN	community psychiatric nurse
CPR	cardiopulmonary resuscitation
CRP	C-reactive protein
CT	computed tomography
CVA	cerebrovascular accident
CXR	chest X-ray
DSM-IV	*Diagnostic and Statistical Manual of Mental Disorders*, 4th edn (Arlington, VA: American Psychiatric Press, 1994)
DSH	deliberate self-harm
ECG	electrocardiography/electrocardiogram
ECT	electroconvulsive therapy
EEG	electroencephalogram
EPSE	extrapyramidal side effects
ESR	erythrocyte sedimentation ratio
FBC	full blood count
FTD	formal thought disorder
GAD	generalised anxiety disorder
GGT	gamma-glutamyltransferase
GMC	General Medical Council
GP	general practitioner

HIV	human immunodeficiency virus
ICD-10	*International Classification of Diseases and Related Health Problems*, 10th revision (Geneva: World Health Organization, 2003)
ICU	intensive care unit
IM	intramuscular
IV	intravenous
JVP	jugular venous pulse
LFTs	liver function tests
MAOI	monoamine oxidase inhibitor
MDMA	3,4-methylenedioxymetamphetamine
MMSE	mini-mental state examination
MRI	magnetic resonance imaging
MS	multiple sclerosis
MSE	mental state examination
NMDA	*N*-methyl-D-aspartate
NMS	neuroleptic malignant syndrome
NSAID	non-steroidal anti-inflammatory drug
OCD	obsessive–compulsive disorder
PD	personality disorder
PRN	pro re nata (when required)
PTSD	post-traumatic stress disorder
RT	rapid tranquilisation
SAD	seasonal affective disorder
SCT	subcutaneous tissue
SD	systematic desensitisation
SHO	senior house officer
SLE	systemic lupus erythematosus
SNRI	serotonin noradrenergic re-uptake inhibitor
SSRI	selective serotonin re-uptake inhibitor
TCA	tricyclic antidepressant
TLE	temporal lobe epilepsy
U&E	urea and electrolytes
UTI	urinary tract infection

OSCE ADVICE

THE EXAM STRUCTURE

There are 12 7-minute stations.
There may be a rest station, but this depends on the examination centre.
You have 1 minute to read the scenario and tasks.
You will then hear a buzzer: walk into the station and perform the tasks.
You have 7 minutes to complete your tasks.
At 6 minutes, a buzzer will sound, reminding you that there is 1 minute left to go
At 7 minutes, a buzzer will sound: you must stop whatever you are doing.
Move on to the next station.

Total examination time: 1 hour and 36 minutes (excluding any rest stations).

Instructions vary in length, and number of tasks will differ between stations.

If you finish early, remain in the station.

Practising OSCEs over will give you an inherent sense of the timings.

EXAMINATION CONTENT

Basic components of history-taking, examination skills (e.g. cranial nerves, motor system, fundal examination), practical skills (e.g. application of ECG leads), emergencies (e.g. resuscitation) and communication skills (e.g. explaining treatment, consent to treatment, prognosis) are all likely to be examined.

MARKING

According to the Royal College of Psychiatrists, a minimum of grade C in at least nine stations is required to pass. Failing any station with grade E (severe fail) means that the candidate fails the OSCE overall (see www.rcpsych.ac.uk/traindev/exams/index.htm). A useful way of revising is to think, at each station that you practise, about what the examiner might have on his or her mark sheet. In our answers, we have included points that we believe the examiner will be marking you on.

OSCE TECHNIQUE

Remember: IEP (I'm an Excellent Psychiatrist).

Introduce yourself to the patient (use their name if given): 'Hello Mrs Jones. My name is Dr Smith.'
Explain what it is you have been asked (or would like) to do and make sure they are okay with this (permission).

Setting the scene is a useful way to start and can give you some thinking time should you require it. For example, 'I'm sorry to hear you've been having side effects from the medication. Would it be alright if you told me how the medication has been affecting you?'

GENERAL ADVICE

- Try to impart information to the patient clearly (this needs practice).
- Clear speech communicates intelligence and competence.
- Speak in lay terms to patients.
- Speak in professional terms in stations where the actor pretends to be a colleague or the tasks directly involve the examiner.
- Start each interview with open questions and then become more focused, e.g. 'Can you tell me how you have been feeling recently?'
- Avoid swing questions, e.g. 'Are you feeling high or low?' – not good.
- Avoid leading questions, e.g. 'You're feeling low now, aren't you?'
- Don't ignore non-verbal signs, e.g. tremor.
- Pauses and moments of silence are acceptable, especially after emotional responses. Be empathetic in such situations.
- Exert control if you find the patient veering off the subject. Bring them back gently to the task you need to complete. 'We were just talking about the voices...' 'To come back to the voices you've been hearing...' 'Could you tell me some more about the voices?'
- It is better to say you don't know something than to make it up. Sometimes, delaying an answer works well. 'I will look into this and get back to you'.
- You must practise doing more than one station at a time so that you learn how to overcome a poor performance in a previous station.
- Although time will often be short, appearing unrushed and calm looks professional.
- Know the ICD-10 diagnostic criteria for the common conditions.
- Think safe and consider the risk element in each station.
- Have a general medical colleague run through physical examinations of the main systems (cardiovascular, etc.) with you so you will feel more confident.

DEMEANOUR

- Body language is very important. Do not slouch, fold your arms or cross your legs. Rather, sit on the chair, with both feet on the ground, leaning slightly towards the actor. Your hands should be together or holding paper.
- Be confident and professional but not arrogant.
- Remaining calm throughout inspires confidence in the examiner.
- Smiling if appropriate shows that you are relaxed and demonstrates confidence.
- Be keen and interested in the patient.

DEALING WITH THE ACTORS

- You are acting as much as they are: you must pretend that all the scenarios are real, otherwise you might underperform.
- Always put the 'patient' at ease.
- Try to develop rapport (supportive remarks).
- Listen to what they are saying to you – don't ignore important cues.
- Actors have been instructed to be difficult or to get upset at certain stations, so don't take it personally; you can score highly if you handle it well.

EXAM DAY

- There have been reports of confusion at the OSCE centres – be prepared for this.
- Be blinkered as you pass through your stations. Don't get distracted by another candidate performing at their station.
- Remember that the candidate before you is direct competition. You must 'up' your performance on exam day.
- Read each station and the set tasks very carefully.
- Most of us are anxious on exam day, but try to settle down quickly. If you are too anxious, the examiner becomes anxious about you (practising will reduce anxiety levels).
- Never dwell on a previous station, even if it seems disastrous. You gave your best shot, so now move on. Failure to do so is likely to damage your concentration and performance in the next one or two stations.
- Don't attempt to read what the examiner might be writing.
- Always thank the patient at the end.
- Talk to the examiner only if instructed to do so or if they speak directly to you. You can acknowledge the examiner at the end of the station if you wish, but don't overdo it.

ISSUES THAT CANDIDATES HAVE RAISED WITH US BEFORE THE EXAM

I'm shy, but I think I know enough to pass: what should I do?

On the day, you must appear confident and speak clearly, so both the examiner and actor can hear you. Practise as much as you can with seniors and colleagues. Some people find it helpful to record their practice sessions using a small cassette recorder and listening back to themselves.

I find it hard to keep to the seven minutes

By practising repeatedly, you will get a good feel for 7 minutes. If possible, do not finish a station too early.

The OSCE is harder to pass than the individual patient assessment

Of course, there are advantages and disadvantages to both. The OSCE tends to examine a broader range of knowledge and skills, unlike the IPA, where small areas can be examined in depth. The important take-home message is that almost the same percentage of people pass the OSCE as passed the IPA. So, do the work and you should pass.

Seven minutes is not enough time to complete the tasks

Remember: the good thing about the OSCE is that there is supposed to be consistency. If time is short for you, then it will be short for everyone. You cannot cover everything in 7 minutes, and an actor might obstruct your interview progress. By practising, you will learn what you can realistically cover for the majority of OSCEs. Know the diagnostic criteria for the main disorders, how to take short focused histories, how to elicit relevant psychopathology, etc. Knowing how to do this by heart will limit time wasted.

What should I do if I finish too early?

This can feel uncomfortable, especially if you have a minute or more remaining. This shouldn't happen if you practise. Stock phrases in this situation can be useful, e.g. 'Do you have any questions for me?' 'We've covered a number of issues. Is there anything else you would like to tell me?'

I get distracted if I hear other candidates doing their OSCE

This skill is fundamental to doing well. You must learn to ignore the noise from other candidates and actors. We have found that by rehearsing several stations alongside each other, you can overcome this problem. This does, however, require five to six people, so it can be difficult to organise. Alternatively, practising with the radio or television on can help.

Should I talk to the examiner whilst I do a physical examination on a patient or present my findings at the end?

This depends on the station instructions. If they state 'Present your findings to the examiner', then that's straightforward. If the instruction is simply 'Examine this patient's lower limbs', then we recommend talking to the patient (for the benefit of the examiner) as you examine them. For example, whilst examining the relevant body part, ask: 'Have you noticed that you've lost muscle bulk in your legs?' 'Has the skin colour changed at all?' 'Have you lost any strength in either leg?'

It's difficult to re-create the OSCE situation in my revision group

It shouldn't be. You need:

A minimum of three in a group (candidate, actor, examiner)
A space with a screen or a door

A stop-clock or watch
A selection of OSCEs

The candidate should do a minimum of two to three stations in a row, followed by the actor and examiner giving feedback. Consider how things could have been done better. Rotate roles.

ISSUES THAT CANDIDATES HAVE RAISED WITH US AFTER THE EXAM

The patient refused to shake my hand when I introduced myself

If this happens at a station, then it is an unwelcome start. There are a number of reasons why a patient might not want to shake hands (withdrawn, psychotic, fear of contamination). We would recommend introducing yourself as described above. If the patient offers a hand, then take it – otherwise don't. You can make a good first impression without shaking hands.

I was surprised we had to examine a thyroid gland

We should be able to perform basic physical examinations in our day-to-day practice already. Brushing up for the purposes of the exam will not be too arduous.

The actor was horrible and shouted at me. I'm going to fail

Never lose sight of the fact that the actors have a script. They are not supposed to stray wildly from this. If they lose their temper with you, they should do this with everyone. Remember: it's 'a show' and you are acting too. Irrespective of the tasks set, you must listen to the patient and remain calm, professional and empathetic. Never argue with the actor!

I was already exhausted halfway through and shattered by the end

The OSCE is tiring. You are exposed fairly rapidly to new scenarios and different faces. There's little time to settle, and your adrenals will be working hard. The more exposure you have to sitting multiple OSCEs before the real exam, then the better prepared and adjusted you will be on the day.

EXAMPLE MARK SHEET

Station Title: Anorexia Nervosa (take a dietary and weight history)

Station Number:

Candidate Number:

Candidate Name:

For each category mark as:
A = excellent, B = good, C = average, D = fail, E = severe fail

	A	B	C	D	E
Communication	❏	❏	❏	❏	❏
Diet history	❏	❏	❏	❏	❏
Weight history	❏	❏	❏	❏	❏
Methods used to lose weight	❏	❏	❏	❏	❏
Thoughts re food and weight	❏	❏	❏	❏	❏
Answering other questions	❏	❏	❏	❏	❏
Global rating	❏	❏	❏	❏	❏

QUICK TOPIC REFERENCE

EXAM 4

Antidepressant discontinuation symptoms
Frontal lobes
Features of alcohol dependence
Bipolar disorder: preventing a relapse
Agoraphobia
Bulimia nervosa
MRI interpretation
Respiratory system
Hypochondriacal disorder
Explaining cognitive behavioural therapy
Grief reaction
Chronic schizophrenia

EXAM 5

Capacity
Lithium advice
Cardiovascular examination
Panic disorder
Parietal lobe assessment
Intoxicated patient
Psychosis
Chronic fatigue syndrome (neurasthenia)
Testamentary capacity
Travel and lithium
X-ray interpretation
Erotomania

EXAM 6

Pregnancy and breastfeeding
Opiate addiction
Data interpretation
Cannabis
Intramuscular injection
Obsessions: assessment
Lower-limb examination
Risk assessment: suicidal patient
Rapid tranquilisation
Seasonal affective disorder
Temporal lobe assessment
SSRIs: sexual dysfunction

EXAM 7

Anorexia nervosa
Perinatal disorder
Perform an ECG
Hazards of injecting illicit drugs
Manic patient
Social phobia
Fundoscopy
Lithium and hypothyroidism
Dementia: wandering
Stopping medication
Personality
Withdrawn behaviour

EXAM 8

Basic life support
Eating disorder
ECG interpretation
Stimulant use
Korsakoff's syndrome
Antidepressant treatment
Hyperprolactinaemia
Risk assessment
Risk assessment: speaking to the consultant on the phone
Neuropsychiatric lupus (SLE)
Delusional jealousy
Liver disease

EXAM 1

STATION 1

The husband of a patient with mild dementia sees you in your outpatient clinic. His wife has had a problem with her memory for some time. He says he has read a little bit about the dementia drugs available but wants you to give him more information.

Provide this gentleman with some information about these medications.

[advice on page 6]

STATION 2

These parents have a 17-year-old daughter recently diagnosed with anorexia nervosa. They had noticed for some time that she would not eat with them at meal times and was losing weight. They have heard of the illness but have a number of questions that they would like to ask.

What are the symptoms of anorexia nervosa?
What is the difference between bulimia and anorexia?
What causes anorexia?
What do you advise we make her eat?

[advice on page 8]

STATION 3

Examine this patient's cranial nerves.

Do not examine: Smell
                    Pinprick to face
                    Gag reflex
                    Corneal reflex

Please use the equipment provided for you.

[advice on page 11]

STATION 4

The mother of a 22-year-old man has asked to see you. Your team has recently diagnosed her son with schizophrenia and she has some questions for you. Before his admission, he had been frankly psychotic and threatening towards her. He thought that MI5 was after him and that his life was in danger. His mother initially did not believe that he was mentally unwell and thought he was using illicit drugs and lazing around. She admits to having been hostile and critical of him and that there were many arguments at home.

She asks you: What is schizophrenia? Is it a split personality?
What will be the effects of the illness on her son?
What are the differences between positive and negative symptoms?
What treatments are available?

[advice on page 14]

STATION 5

A 30-year-old man who was given haloperidol for acute management of a psychotic episode is noticed by nursing staff to be drifting in and out of consciousness on your ward. On further examination, he appears to be quite rigid and pyrexial. He is also tachycardic (pulse 150/min) and hypertensive (blood pressure 210/100 mm Hg).

You have paged the medical specialist registrar, who is now on the telephone.

Explain your preferred diagnosis from the information given above.

He asks you: What might be the differential diagnosis?
What are the clinical features of this condition?
How do you think he should be managed?
What investigations would be useful?
What are the possible medical complications in this case?

[advice on page 17]

STATION 6

Take a history of temporal lobe epilepsy from this patient who takes dothiepin (dosulepin).

[advice on page 20]

STATION 7

A 22-year-old student presents to the outpatients' department. He is in a wheelchair and reports being unable to walk. On examination, he has normal reflexes in his lower limbs. Several physicians have been unable to identify a neurological cause.

Take a history for a possible neurotic cause and present your findings to the examiner.

[advice on page 23]

STATION 8

This patient has been on amitriptyline for some time. He remains depressed.

Discuss lithium augmentation with this man.

[advice on page 25]

STATION 9

Discuss the treatment of obsessive–compulsive disorder with this patient.

[advice on page 27]

STATION 10

A 40-year-old woman with a diagnosis of schizophrenia has had a recent florid psychotic episode. She drives her children to school every day.

Advise her about driving.

[advice on page 29]

STATION 11

This woman has a diagnosis of agoraphobia. She becomes extremely anxious when faced with the prospect of having to leave the house.

Explain desensitisation therapy for agoraphobia.

[advice on page 31]

STATION 12

Carry out a risk assessment on this male patient who has taken an overdose.

[advice on page 33]

STATION 1: DEMENTIA MEDICATION

THE EXAMINER'S MARK SHEET	
Communication skills	Treatments available
Empathy	Answering other questions
Risks/benefits	Global rating

INTRODUCE YOURSELF

'Hello, nice to meet you. My name is Dr Smith.'

SET THE SCENE

'I understand that you would like to know some more about the drugs currently available for dementia. Is this correct?'

FIND OUT WHAT HE ALREADY KNOWS

'Would it be OK to ask you what you already know about these medications?'
Always find out how much someone knows before assuming they know nothing.

INFORMATION ON MEDICATION

Use lay terms. Allow the husband to interrupt with questions if he has any.
Explain that the drugs do not represent a cure for dementia but are thought to delay the course of the disease.

Ask whether he knows which form of dementia his wife has been diagnosed with (e.g. Alzheimer's, vascular, Lewy body, mixed) and who made the diagnosis (specialist or GP).

'The medications available currently are the acetylcholinesterase (AChE) inhibitors (AIs) and memantine.'

'Three AIs (donepezil, galantamine, rivastigmine) are currently available. They are all very similar in their clinical effects on memory and improved attention and motivation.'

'It is not entirely clear how long someone can continue to benefit from these medicines, but some degree of cognitive improvement may be evident for 9–12 months and often they are taken for several years. Usually, if no improvement is noticed after 3–4 months, then the medication is stopped. They are usually tolerated well, although side effects can include nausea, vomiting, reduced appetite, diarrhoea, tiredness, poor sleep and headache.'

'AIs work by reducing the breakdown of acetylcholine, an important brain transmitter. The level of acetylcholine in the brain is reduced significantly in Alzheimer's disease. These drugs increase the presence of acetylcholine in the brain and modify some of the effects of dementia, such as poor memory, at least temporarily. Research has shown that approximately 50 per cent of patients with dementia who are prescribed these medications can improve or stabilise over a 6-month period [NICE 2001 guidelines: see below].'

'Memantine is a medication used for treating moderate to severe Alzheimer's disease. It is from a different family of medication to the AIs. Your wife is mildly affected, so we would not consider this medication currently.'

ASK WHETHER HE HAS ANY QUESTIONS

THANK HIM

FOR EXTRA MARKS

National Institute for Clinical Excellence (NICE) guidelines on the use of donepezil, rivastigmine and galantamine for Alzheimer's disease (January 2001):

MMSE score of 12 or above.
Confirmation of Alzheimer's disease in a specialist clinic.
The patient must be likely to take their medication.
Treatment must be started in a specialist setting following assessment.
Assessment should be repeated 2–4 months after reaching maintenance dose.
Patients who continue on the drug should be assessed every 6 months.

These guidelines are overdue for re-review so may change in the near future.

Donepezil is a reversible inhibitor of AChE and is taken once daily.
Galantamine is a reversible inhibitor of AChE and has nicotinic receptor agonist properties.
Rivastigmine is a reversible non-competitive inhibitor of AChE.

A recent randomised study suggested that donepezil was not cost-effective, with benefits below minimally relevant thresholds. The authors of this study recommended that more effective treatments than cholinesterase inhibitors were needed for Alzheimer's disease (*Lancet* 2004; **363**: 2100–1).

However, small improvements in cognitive and global assessments in Alzheimer's disease with cholinesterase inhibitors have only ever been claimed.

Memantine is an NMDA receptor antagonist affecting glutamate transmission. This drug has been used in Germany for over a decade.

FURTHER READING

Evans JG, Wilcock G, Birks J. Evidence based pharmacotherapy of Alzheimer's disease. *Int J Neuropsychopharmacol* 2004; **7**: 35–69.
Rogawski MA, Wenk GL. The neuropharmacological basis for the use of memantine in the treatment of Alzheimer's disease. *CNS Drug Rev* 2003; **9**: 275–308.

STATION 2: ANOREXIA NERVOSA

THE EXAMINER'S MARK SHEET

Communication skills	Aetiology
Symptoms of AN	Dietary advice
Differences between AN and BN	Global rating

INTRODUCE YOURSELF

'Hello, nice to meet you. My name is Dr Smith.'

SET THE SCENE

'I understand your daughter has recently been diagnosed with anorexia nervosa and you have a number of questions for me. Is that correct?'

FIND OUT WHAT THEY ALREADY KNOW

'Would it be OK to ask you what you already know about anorexia nervosa?'

INFORMATION ON ANOREXIA NERVOSA

Symptoms

Fear of fatness
Undereating
Excessive loss of weight
Increased exercise
Monthly periods stop

'You may have noticed your daughter missing meals, eating little, avoiding eating in public, believing she is too fat, exercising frequently, using the bathroom after meals, vomiting or using laxatives.'

Differences between bulimia and anorexia

Bulimia: Fear of fatness
          Binge-eating
          Vomiting/purging/use of laxatives
          Normal weight (often also underweight)
          Irregular periods

Many young women want to be slimmer and more attractive, even if they are not overweight. Sometimes, despite being of normal weight, the need to be slimmer becomes an obsession, which can lead to problems. In AN, worries tend to be about weight, which leads to a dramatic restriction in nutritional intake. Whilst someone with BN also worries about their weight, they switch between limiting their nutritional intake and eating to excess in short periods of time (bingeing). They commonly induce vomiting or use laxatives to limit weight gain.

Aetiology

A number of important factors are thought to be involved:

Social: media, fashion, advertising, peers, popular diets.

Control: weight loss can lead to a sense of control when other areas of the patient's life feel out of control.

Puberty: extreme weight loss can delay puberty and sexual development; the demands of maturing and growing up therefore can be delayed.

Family: refusing food at meal times can exert control in family interactions; eating disorders can run in families.

Life events: AN can be triggered by a traumatic episode such as a bereavement or the divorce of one's parents.

Dietary advice

It is common for children with AN to resent their parents trying to interfere with their eating, and such pressure may worsen the situation. The person may respond better to the advice of someone outside the family, such as an eating disorders specialist or the family doctor. If she has not already been referred to a specialist, then this should be recommended.

The Royal College of Psychiatrists advises the following:

Eat regular meals, including breakfast, lunch and dinner.

Eat a balanced diet.

Include carbohydrates with each meal.

Don't skip meals.

Avoid sugary and high-fat snacks.

Take regular exercise.

Try not to be influenced by other people skipping meals or commenting on weight.

Offer the parents some information leaflets about the disorder.

ASK WHETHER THEY HAVE ANY OTHER QUESTIONS

THANK THEM

FOR EXTRA MARKS

You would want to see and assess their daughter. Who made the diagnosis?
She may need referral to a specialist service. What is her BMI?
You must know the ICD-10 criteria for AN and BN.
If the illness is causing medical ill health, then she will need to see the
medical team urgently.
Know the common physical signs and biochemical changes that occur.
This is a serious illness (it carries the highest mortality of any mental illness).
It is important to be honest but tactful if this comes up.
Know about good/bad prognostic indicators.

SUPPORT GROUPS/ADVICE

Eating Disorders Association: www.edauk.com
YoungMinds: www.youngminds.org.uk
Schmidt U, Treasure J. *Getting Better Bit(e) by Bit(e): A Survival Kit for
Sufferers of Bulimia Nervosa and Binge Eating Disorders*. London: Psychology
Press, 1993.

FURTHER READING

Walsh BT, Klein DA. Eating disorders. *Int Rev Psychiatry* 2003; **15**: 205–16.

STATION 3: CRANIAL NERVES EXAMINATION

THE EXAMINER'S MARK SHEET	
Communication skills	Technique
Approach to patient	Answering other questions
CN II to XII examined	Global rating

INTRODUCE YOURSELF

'Hello, nice to meet you. My name is Dr Smith.'

SET THE SCENE

'I have been asked to examine you. This will involve some simple tests, including looking at your eyes and testing your hearing.'

ASK FOR PERMISSION

'Would that be OK?'
'Let me know if you are uncomfortable at any point.'

CLINICAL PROCEDURE

The patient should be sitting.
As in all clinical examinations, ideally you should be on the patient's right-hand side.

CN I

'Do you have any problems with your sense of *smell*?' (Asked not to do here.)

CN II

'Do you have any problems with your *eyesight*?'
Ask them to put on their glasses if they normally wear them.
'Can you see that clock on the wall [or similar distant object]?'
'What does it say?'

Visual fields: Use your finger or red-headed pin if available.
'Keep looking at my nose' – ask the subject to cover one eye.
'Tell me when you see the pin' – map out their field of vision.

Fundoscopy: see Exam 7, Station 7.

CN III, IV, VI

Light reflex and accommodation:	convergence reflex (with your finger close to the subject's nose, ask them to look at an object in the distance and then at your finger).
Eye movements:	'Can you see my finger? Keep looking at it whilst it moves' (move in the shape of a cross).

At the extremes of their gaze, ask whether they can see one or two fingers (i.e. double vision). Also look for nystagmus.

CN VII

Facial movement: 'Raise your eyebrows, screw up your eyes tightly, puff out your cheeks, whistle, show me your teeth.'

CN V

'Clench your teeth' – as they do, feel masseter and temporalis.
'Open your mouth and stop me closing it' – try gently to close the chin.

CN IX, X

Palate and gag reflex: 'Open your mouth and say aah' – look at back of throat (gag reflex – touch back of throat both sides with an orange stick – but asked not to do here).

CN XII

Tongue: Ask patient to stick out tongue. Observe for deviation to left/right. Observe resting tongue for wasting and fasciculation.

CN XI

Accessory nerve: 'Shrug your shoulders and don't let me push them down.'
'Turn your head to the right ...' (feel their left sternomastoid)
'... and to the left' (feel right side).

CN VIII

Hearing: 'How is your hearing?'
Can they hear you rubbing your index finger against your thumb in each ear?

CN V

Trigeminal – sensation: 'Can you feel when I touch here?' Use finger/cotton wool. Examine ophthalmic, maxillary and mandibular territories of their face (corneal reflex – not to test here).

THANK THE PATIENT

FOR EXTRA MARKS

You will often be asked to omit pinprick, corneal and gag testing, but be able to do them in practice.

It is possible to assess all nerves within 7 minutes.

REMEMBER:

Smell and taste (I, VII, IX)
Visual acuity (II)
Visual field (II)
Eye movements (III, IV, VI)
Nystagmus (VIII and cerebellum)
Ptosis (III, sympathetic)
Pupils (III)
Discs (II)
Facial movements (V, VII)
Palatal movements (IX, X)
Gag reflex (IX, X)
Tongue (XII)
Accessory (XI)
Hearing (VIII)
Facial sensation (V)
Corneal reflex (V)

FURTHER READING

www.neuroexam.com
http://medlib.med.utah.edu/neurologicexam/home_exam.html

STATION 4: SCHIZOPHRENIA

THE EXAMINER'S MARK SHEET	
Communication skills	Positive and negative symptoms
Schizophrenia explanation	Treatments available
Effects on her son	Global rating

INTRODUCE YOURSELF

'Hello, nice to meet you. My name is Dr Smith.'

SET THE SCENE

'Thank you for coming to see me. I understand you have some questions about schizophrenia. Is that correct?'

FIND OUT WHAT THEY ALREADY KNOW

'Would it be OK to ask you what you already know about schizophrenia?'

INFORMATION ON SCHIZOPHRENIA

Remember to speak in lay terms. Be empathetic.

What is schizophrenia?

'Schizophrenia is a serious mental illness. It affects about one in every 100 people and usually comes to light in the late teens or early adult life. Thinking, emotions and behaviour are often affected. Unusual behaviour may include delusions, hallucinations and/or a lack of insight.'

Ask whether they know what these terms mean. If not, then explain them.

'Generally speaking, around one-quarter of affected people make a reasonable recovery, but for others it can be a lifelong illness and can be quite disabling.'

Is it a split personality?

'Many people believe this from what they have heard in the media, but this is a common misunderstanding.'

What are the differences between positive and negative symptoms?

'The symptoms of schizophrenia can be divided into two groups for convenience, called positive and negative symptoms. Not everyone affected will experience all of the possible symptoms.'

Positive symptoms include delusions, thought disorder and hallucinations:

Delusions are strongly held beliefs that are unusual and false. Often, no amount of persuasion will convince the person otherwise.

Thought disorder is a disturbance of thought processes. Sentences may make little or no sense, words may be used inappropriately and new words may be made up.

Hallucinations are experiences of hearing, seeing, feeling or smelling things that are not actually there. They feel very real and can be frightening to the person experiencing them. They make some people feel vulnerable and suspicious of others.

Negative symptoms usually occur in chronic schizophrenia after a number of years. Individuals become quiet and withdrawn and appear unemotional. Loss of drive, lack of interest in things and lack of motivation are common features; often there is also deterioration in the person's level of personal care.

What will be the effects of this illness on my son?
'Of course, everyone is individual and some people do much better than others. In our experience, people with schizophrenia often have difficulties with . . .'

Work (often difficult to commit to the demands of employment)
Socialising, e.g. maintaining relationships
Depression (low mood and suicidal thoughts are common)
Low self-esteem

What treatments are available?
'Firstly, the earlier and quicker someone is diagnosed and treated, the better.'
'Some people make a full recovery.'
Discuss the importance of the following and their roles in management:

Medication
The multidisciplinary team
Family
Day centres and work projects
Psychotherapy (targeted at abnormal perceptions or mood symptoms)
Organisations: Rethink, Mind, SANE

ASK WHETHER SHE HAS ANY OTHER QUESTIONS

THANK HER

FOR EXTRA MARKS

Be prepared for relatives to be upset and angry. Remain calm and empathetic. Whatever happens, do not get angry with them, even if you think you are failing the station.

People with schizophrenia are rarely dangerous.
One in four people with schizophrenia will get better within the first 5 years.

SUPPORT GROUPS/ADVICE

Mind (National Association for Mental Health): www.mind.org.uk
Rethink (National Schizophrenia Fellowship): www.rethink.org
SANE: www.sane.org.uk
Royal College of Psychiatrists: www.rcpsych.ac.uk
www.schizophrenia.com

STATION 5: NEUROLEPTIC MALIGNANT SYNDROME

INTRODUCE YOURSELF

SET THE SCENE

'Thank you for answering your pager. I'm very concerned about a 30-year-old patient on our ward who is acutely unwell following a dose of haloperidol that we have given him. I believe he has a likely neuroleptic malignant syndrome (NMS) and would be grateful if you could assess him urgently.'

FIND OUT WHAT THEY ALREADY KNOW

'Thankfully, we don't see NMS as often these days. Have you ever seen a case yourself? Do you know much about it?'

INFORMATION ON NMS

Differential diagnosis

Neurological: infection, neoplasia, cerebrovascular disease, head trauma, seizures

Systemic: infection, metabolic diseases, endocrine (e.g. thyrotoxicosis, phaeochromocytoma), SLE

Drugs: alcohol withdrawal, stimulants

Clinical features

Increased body temperature (hyperpyrexia)
Autonomic instability
Altered mental state (always)
Muscular rigidity
Diaphoresis
Sialorrhoea and dysphagia (often)

Management

This is a *medical emergency.*
Patient needs transfer to medical ward or ICU.
Withdraw any antipsychotic medication immediately.

General supportive measures

Keep cool: give antipyretic, use cooling blanket

IV access: take bloods, rehydration with fluids, correct electrolyte imbalances

Hypertension: give antihypertensive

Oxygen

Suction if needed

Pharmacological treatment:

–   dantrolene (muscle relaxant)

–   bromocriptine (dopamine agonist)

–   benzodiazepines

–   prop–ranolol

ECT

Seek senior/expert advice

Investigations

Raised white cell count

Raised LFTs

Raised CPK (can be up to 100 000/L)

Myoglobinuria

Complications

Renal: rhabdomyolysis, leading to renal failure

Cardiovascular: arrhythmias, cardiac arrest, CVA, cardiogenic shock

Respiratory: respiratory failure, pulmonary embolus

Coma

Death

ASK WHETHER HE HAS ANY OTHER QUESTIONS

THANK HIM

FOR EXTRA MARKS

Avoid using lay terms when speaking with colleagues.

RISK FACTORS FOR NMS

Age <20 years or >60 years
CNS dysfunction
Male : female 2 : 1
High neuroleptic dose, rapid neuroleptisation, depot, more than one neuroleptic prescribed
Dehydration, electrolyte disturbance
Previous NMS

TREATMENT OF HIS PSYCHOSIS IN THE FUTURE

At least 5–14-day drug holiday
Rechallenge with structurally different neuroleptic
Start with low dose and titrate slowly
No depot

ASSOCIATED INCIDENCE AND MORTALITY

Incidence one per cent (0.02–2.5 per cent often quoted)
Mortality ten per cent

FURTHER READING

Bhanushauli MJ, Tuite PJ. The evaluation and management of patients with NMS. *Neurol Clin* 2004; 22: 389–411.

STATION 6: TEMPORAL LOBE EPILEPSY

THE EXAMINER'S MARK SHEET	
Communication skills	Medication history
Empathy	Answering other questions
History of temporal lobe epilepsy (TLE) and associated features	Global rating

INTRODUCE YOURSELF

'Hello, nice to meet you. My name is Dr Smith.'

SET THE SCENE

'I understand you have had some seizures. Is that correct?'
'I wanted to find out what happens to you during these episodes.'

ASK FOR PERMISSION

'Would that be OK?'

TAKE A HISTORY OF TEMPORAL LOBE EPILEPSY: KEY AREAS

Details of seizures

What happens?
What do witnesses say?
How long have they been happening, how often, and how long do they last?
Disruption to normal functioning/daily life?

Medication history

What other medications are they taking?
Relationship of seizures to dothiepin (dosulepin) (onset, increased frequency of seizures, higher dose).

Tricyclic antidepressants lower the convulsive threshold.

Family history

Medical history

Head injury, other medical conditions, alcohol or drug misuse, febrile convulsions.
Ask about **interictal periods** (TLE associated with psychosis).

Auras are common: Autonomic effects and visceral sensations
Altered perceptual experiences
Déjà vu and jamais vu
Lilliputian hallucinations
Olfactory and gustatory hallucinations
Cognitive abnormalities (speech, thought, memory)
Strong affective experiences (commonly fear/anxiety)

TEST TEMPORAL LOBE FUNCTION

Only if time allows.

Dominant lobe

Receptive dysphasia
Alexia: ask them to read something
Agraphia: ask them to write something
Impaired learning and retention of verbal material: ask them to repeat an address
– '42 West Register Street' – and to recall it after 5 minutes

Non-dominant lobe

Visuospatial difficulties
Anomia: ask them to name a wristwatch, strap and buckle
Prosopagnosia: ask them whether they recognise Queen Elizabeth on a £5 note
Hemisomatopagnosia: belief that a limb is absent, even though it is not
Impaired learning and retention of non-verbal material, such as music and
drawings: ask them to copy a drawing (see below) and to repeat from memory
5 minutes later

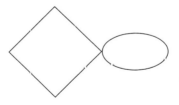

Bilateral lesions

Amnesic syndromes (Korsakoff's amnesia, Klüver–Bucy syndrome): assess short-
and long-term memories.

ASK WHETHER THE PATIENT HAS ANY QUESTIONS

THANK THE PATIENT

FOR EXTRA MARKS

Consequences of neurological damage to temporal lobe structures: changes in behaviour/personality.

Enquire about change in themselves: increased aggression, agitation or instability (limbic system).

Assess visual fields: contralateral homonymous upper quadrantanopia.

Other:

depersonalisation

disturbance of sexual function

epileptic phenomena

psychotic disturbances akin to schizophrenia

FURTHER READING

Ojensann GA. Treatment of temporal lobe epilepsy. *Annu Rev Med* 1997; 48: 317–28.

STATION 7: CONVERSION DISORDER

THE EXAMINER'S MARK SHEET	
Communication skills	Precipitants/life events
Empathy	Relevant mental state examination
History of deficit	Global rating

INTRODUCE YOURSELF

'Hello, nice to meet you. My name is Dr Smith.'

SET THE SCENE

'I'm sorry to learn that you have had some problems with walking. I wanted to talk to you about this.'

ASK FOR PERMISSION

'Would that be OK?'

TAKE A HISTORY OF CONVERSION DISORDER: KEY AREAS

Take a history that demonstrates to the examiner that conversion disorder is the most likely diagnosis.

History of presenting complaint

Ask about the temporal sequence of events involved with the reported paralysis. Was there a sudden onset of symptoms in clear relation to stress?

'That must have been very difficult when you lost the use of your lower limbs.'
'Can you tell me about your life at that time?'
'Had there been any changes or events out of the ordinary?'

What is the patient's understanding of events/beliefs?
Why has no physical cause has been identified?
Symptoms can be somewhat variable in comparison with organic symptoms, where they tend to be consistent.
Ask questions to show you have considered a hypochondriacal or somatisation disorder. Try to elicit evidence of primary and secondary gain.

Past psychiatric history

Previous episodes.
Past presentations to hospital or general practitioner.

ASK WHETHER HE HAS ANY QUESTIONS

THANK HIM

NOTE

As conversion disorder becomes less common in clinical practice (*Psychol Med* 1975; 5: 9–12), one would have thought it would be less likely to feature in an exam. Examiners can, however, have a soft spot for the more dramatic expressions of mental illness. From this point of view, conversion disorder fits the bill.

The central feature of conversion disorder is a loss of function that appears to be due to a physical cause but is in fact due to an underlying psychological conflict.

FOR EXTRA MARKS

Do not get into an argument about the origins of symptoms.

The actor might ask you about the origin of the symptoms in conversion disorder, e.g. 'What is causing these problems doctor?' The best response is to say: 'There is a disconnection between the mind and the more external parts of the body following a recent stressful event.'

There will usually have been extensive investigations ruling out a physical cause, so it is unwise to support any discussion about a physical cause.

Suggest that you would have liked to have examined the lower limbs.

Definitive diagnosis of dissociative (conversion) disorder requires no evidence of physical cause and sufficient knowledge of the psychological, social and personal relationships of the patient to formulate a dissociative aetiology (ICD-10).

FURTHER READING

Lewis A. The survival of hysteria. *Psychol Med* 1975; 5: 9–12.

STATION 8: LITHIUM AUGMENTATION

THE EXAMINER'S MARK SHEET	
Communication skills	Adverse effects
Lithium explanation	Answering other questions
Risks/benefits	Global rating

INTRODUCE YOURSELF

'Hello, nice to meet you. My name is Dr Smith.'

SET THE SCENE

'I understand that you've been on the antidepressant amitriptyline for some time now. Is that right?'

'Sometimes, when antidepressants don't work as much as we had hoped, adding in a treatment called lithium can help.'

FIND OUT WHAT THEY ALREADY KNOW

'Have you heard of lithium?'

'What do you know about lithium treatment?'

INFORMATION ON LITHIUM

Reasons for considering adding lithium

Lithium appears to be associated with an acute antidepressant effect in up to 50 per cent of patients otherwise refractory to monotherapy.

In situations where single medications do not seem to have an effect, lithium has been shown to be useful as an additional medication to treat depression.

Three major issues to consider

Caution about side effects.

Warn about lithium toxicity.

Describe lithium treatment and the need for plasma level monitoring (blood testing).

Pre-lithium work-up

Baseline investigation of renal function

ECG

Thyroid function tests

'Because lithium is eliminated by the kidneys, it is important to check how well the kidneys are working by performing a renal function test before starting any lithium therapy.'

'Because lithium can interfere with thyroid function, we like to check the thyroid before we start treatment, and then 6-monthly thereafter. We also take a tracing of the heart to confirm that there are no pre-existing abnormalities that may worsen with lithium treatment.'

A concentration of 0.5–1.0 mmol/L is usually sufficient for clinical effect. Because the dose has to be kept within certain limits, the blood has to be monitored initially after 5–7 days, and then weekly until the correct level has been reached. Finally, levels should be monitored every 3–6 months when stabilisation has occurred.

Lithium is prescribed as a single dose at night.

ASK WHETHER HE HAS ANY QUESTIONS

THANK HIM

FOR EXTRA MARKS

The most common side effects are tremor, polyuria, weight gain and nausea.
The tremor can sometimes be treated with a beta-blocker.
The nausea can be counteracted by taking the lithium with food; sometimes, changing the preparation of lithium can make a difference.
Mention interactions with other drugs, e.g. diuretics, NSAIDs, haloperidol.
Offer a patient information leaflet.

FURTHER READING

Ferrier IN, Tyrer SP, Bell AJ. Lithium therapy. *Adv Psychiatr Treat* 1995; 1: 102–10.
Shelton RC The use of antidepressants in novel combination therapies. *J Clin Psychiatry* 2003; 64 (Suppl 2): 14–18.

STATION 9: OBSESSIVE–COMPULSIVE DISORDER

THE EXAMINER'S MARK SHEET	
Communication skills	Pharmacological treatment
Empathy	Answering other questions
Psychological treatment	Global rating

INTRODUCE YOURSELF

'Hello, nice to meet you. My name is Dr Smith.'

SET THE SCENE

'I've been asked to talk to you about the treatments available for obsessive–compulsive disorder (OCD).'

FIND OUT WHAT THEY ALREADY KNOW

'Can I start by asking you what you already know about OCD?'
'Do you know any of the treatments available and what they involve?'
'Have you had treatment yourself in the past? What was this?'

INFORMATION ON OCD TREATMENT

Management

A combination of psychological and pharmacological therapies is probably the most effective approach. (It is appropriate to gauge the nature, e.g. thoughts and/or acts, and the severity of the illness before discussing any management with this patient.)

Reassurance is a key component in the management of OCD. OCD is not a condition that goes away overnight – it is usually chronic and fluctuating.

Exposure and response prevention

Performing rituals can relieve anxiety, but in general the more the rituals are performed, the worse the patient gets. Therefore, it is important to reduce the number of rituals performed.

Exposure must occur for the patient to feel anxiety and want to perform the ritual. This is done by, for example, having the patient touch public handrails or door-handles and then preventing them from washing their hands.

The response prevention is the tricky bit, and in reality anything that will work in practice will be used. This may include verbal coaxing and persuasion, distraction, and performing or engaging in alternative behaviour.

Family members and friends can be enlisted as therapeutic allies. However, at all stages it is important to avoid *conflict*. This only causes setbacks.

Modelling is a technique whereby, for example, the therapist touches handrails or door-handles and then engages in alternative activities. The therapist is setting an example for the patient to do the same thing and not engage in rituals. Modelling is not more effective than exposure and response prevention.

Pharmacological agents
Clomipramine – potent serotonin reuptake inhibitor
SSRIs (serotonin thought to help with obsessional symptoms)

ASK WHETHER THE PATIENT HAS ANY QUESTIONS

THANK THE PATIENT

FOR EXTRA MARKS

CLOMIPRAMINE
Any depressive symptoms are thought to be treated by the main metabolite *n*-desmethylclomipramine.
Takes more than 4 weeks to be effective.
If OCD is severe, then start with clomipramine or an SSRI to reduce the obsessional behaviour. Then implement a psychological programme of exposure and response prevention.
Generally, response to antidepressants takes longer in OCD than in depression.

FURTHER READING
Goodman WK. Obsessive–compulsive disorder: diagnosis and treatment. *J Clin Psychiatry* 1999; **60** (Suppl 18): 27–32.

STATION 10: DRIVING AND THE DVLA

THE EXAMINER'S MARK SHEET	
Communication skills	Basic DVLA rules
Empathy	Answering other questions
Risks of driving	Global rating

INTRODUCE YOURSELF

'Hello, nice to meet you. My name is Dr Smith.'

SET THE SCENE

'I wanted to talk to you about driving. Would that be OK?'

FIND OUT WHAT SHE ALREADY KNOWS

'Have you ever had to contact the DVLA about driving your car?'
'Do you know anything about the DVLA rules and driving, having recently been unwell?'

INFORMATION ON DRIVING AND MENTAL ILLNESS

Try to determine from the patient:

Whether she remains unwell.
If she is still unwell, how long this has been for.

If the patient has been free from the acute psychotic episode for more than 3 months and she is now well, then she is likely to be able to drive with a psychiatric report and DVLA approval.
If 3 months have not elapsed and the patient is still unwell, then it is unlikely that the patient will be allowed to drive.
If the medication taken affects driving performance, then this will influence a DVLA decision. Ask what medication she takes.
Express concerns with regard to her children if she is unfit to drive.

Basic DVLA guidelines

The DVLA states that driving must cease during the acute illness.
The driving licence is reissued when the patient has remained well and stable for at least 3 months, is compliant with treatment, is free from the adverse effects of medication, and obtains a 'favourable specialist report'.
This is not fixed at 3 months for everybody: patients with marked instability will be disallowed from driving for longer periods.
In the case of continuing symptoms, the DVLA is less clear. It states that a patient may even have limited insight and still be allowed to drive as long as the

symptoms do not cause significant concentration problems, memory impairment or distraction.

It is the DVLA's decision as to whether the person is allowed to drive.

It is important to let her know that driving without permission from the DVLA is illegal and that any car insurance is likely to be invalid.

ASK WHETHER SHE HAS ANY QUESTIONS

THANK HER

FOR EXTRA MARKS

In reality, many patients drive while unwell and even during the acute phase of illness. In many instances, this goes unnoticed; however, it can be extremely dangerous.

The question arises as to who is responsible for the patient's actions while driving. The answer is that it is the patient's responsibility to inform the DVLA of their illness. If the clinician feels, however, that the patient has not informed the DVLA, then it is the clinician's duty to make sure that the patient does so. In some cases, the clinician has to inform the DVLA to protect the public and, in this case, the patient's children.

When a patient has a condition that makes driving unsafe and the patient is either unable to appreciate this or refuses to cease driving, then GMC guidelines advise breaking confidentiality and informing the DVLA: www.gmc-uk.org/standards/default.htm.

FURTHER READING

www.dvla.gov.uk/at_a_glance/ch4_psychiatric.htm

STATION 11: EXPLAINING DESENSITISATION THERAPY

THE EXAMINER'S MARK SHEET	
Communication skills	Answering other questions
Empathy	Global rating
Therapy explanation	

INTRODUCE YOURSELF

'Hello, nice to meet you. My name is Dr Smith.'

SET THE SCENE

'I'm sorry to hear it's been very difficult for you recently, particularly when trying to leave your home. I wanted to talk to you about a treatment called desensitisation.'

FIND OUT WHAT SHE ALREADY KNOWS

'Do you know anything about systematic desensitisation (SD)?'

INFORMATION ON DESENSITISATION THERAPY

Start by differentiating between psychological and pharmacological therapy: 'SD is a psychological therapy, meaning that medications are not used for this type of treatment.'

SD is a method of treatment in which the patient is trained to relax in the presence of increasingly fearful situations. If, as described, the agoraphobia is centred around being unable to leave the house, then explain what the therapy will generally entail:

'This treatment is aimed at helping with your difficulty leaving the house. You will have an assigned therapist who is usually a doctor, psychologist or nurse.'

'It involves reducing your difficulty in very small, controlled steps. This will mean leaving the house in small, bit-by-bit steps.'

'The first step is to imagine leaving the house in your mind. Then relaxation is practised when anxiety is experienced. Doing this can be useful so that when you actually face the situation, you'll feel that it's a familiar scene that you've already been through successfully.'

'By exposing you to the situation in a supported way with the therapist present, a little bit at a time, you never let yourself get overly anxious. Often, an anxiety hierarchy is used, where you can describe how anxious you feel on a scale of one to ten, one being slightly anxious and ten being extremely anxious.'

'By gradually facing the feared situation and relaxing in between, your mind can't remember having a "bad" experience in any given place, and therefore you'll be more likely to return.'

Listening to relaxation tapes or using breathing techniques before going out can also lessen anxiety. Family members or close friends can sometimes help with the process, occasionally taking the place of the therapist.

ASK WHETHER SHE HAS ANY QUESTIONS

THANK HER

FOR EXTRA MARKS

When SD is conducted in imagination, the session usually lasts about 40 minutes. The overall number of sessions varies widely (average 11) depending on the progress made by the patient.

LIKELY QUESTIONS FROM THE PATIENT

Q: 'Is it possible to continue taking medication while I have this treatment?'

A: 'Yes, you can be on medication while you are receiving this psychological treatment.'

Q: 'How long does this treatment take?'

A: 'It can take just a few sessions or sometimes longer, up to a few months, depending on how much progress is made in the sessions.'

FURTHER READING

Jacobson E. *Progressive Relaxation.* Chicago: University of Chicago Press, 1938.

Wolpe J. *Psychotherapy by Reciprocal Inhibition.* Stanford: Stanford University Press, 1958.

STATION 12: RISK ASSESSMENT: MALE OVERDOSE

THE EXAMINER'S MARK SHEET	
Communication skills	Risk assessment
Empathy	Answering other questions
Overdose details	Global rating

INTRODUCE YOURSELF

'Hello, nice to meet you. My name is Dr Smith.'

SET THE SCENE

'I've been told that you have taken an overdose of medication. Is that right?'
'I was hoping we could talk about the events leading up to this.'

ASK FOR PERMISSION

'Would that be OK?'

RISK ASSESSMENT: KEY AREAS

You must determine all the details surrounding the overdose, i.e.

Where was the overdose taken?
When was the overdose taken?
Who (if anyone) was with them?
What precautions did they take to avoid discovery?

Other important factors

Final act (was a note left?)/suicidal intent.
Social circumstances.
Socioeconomic factors, e.g. unemployment, adverse life events.
Interpersonal difficulties, e.g. arguments with a partner.
Previous violence and/or suicidal behaviour (other high-risk methods).
Evidence of 'rootlessness' or 'social restlessness', e.g. few relationships, frequent changes of address or employment – these are indicators of increased risk.
Presence of a psychiatric disorder associated with increased suicide risk.
Evidence of poor compliance with treatment or disengagement from psychiatric aftercare.
Substance/alcohol misuse or other potential disinhibiting factors, e.g. social background promoting violence.
Identification of any precipitants.

Any changes in mental state or behaviour that have occurred before the incident and/or relapse.

Presence of chronic/painful medical illness.

ASK WHETHER HE HAS ANY QUESTIONS

THANK HIM

FOR EXTRA MARKS

Deliberate self-harm (DSH) is a very important predictor of suicide.

10 to 14 per cent of people who harm themselves eventually kill themselves.

Higher DSH rates in females and between the ages of 15 and 44 years.

90 per cent of all hospital presentations of DSH are with self-poisoning.

Clinical experience indicates that males who self-harm are marginalised, engaging in petty crime, excessive alcohol consumption and irregular employment.

FURTHER READING

Szmukler G. Risk assessment: 'numbers' and 'values'. *Psychiatr Bull* 2003; 27: 205–7.

EXAM 2

STATION 1

This man is an outpatient and has a diagnosis of schizophrenia. He has tried a number of typical and atypical neuroleptics over the past 5 years, but he remains unwell and disturbed by abnormal perceptions. His disturbed mental state has meant that it has been difficult for him to mix with other people or find work.

In his latest medical review, the team have decided to try him on clozapine, if he agrees.

Your consultant asks you to explain this to him and what this involves in terms of risks and benefits.

[advice on page 40]

STATION 2

This 32-year-old woman has a 7-year history of schizophrenia. She was given olanzapine 9 months ago after she complained of extrapyramidal side effects with a typical neuroleptic. She has put on over 4 kg in weight since taking olanzapine. She has concerns that she now looks unattractive and wants to stop her medication.

She wants to know: Why has she put on so much weight with olanzapine?
                     Can she stop the medication?

[advice on page 42]

STATION 3

Examine this patient's abdomen.

[advice on page 44]

STATION 4

This patient has been on lithium treatment for 20 years for bipolar affective disorder. He has tolerated the drug well and his mental state has been stable. He noticed that his neck looked larger when looking through some photographs from a recent party.

Examine this patient's thyroid gland.

Do not take a psychiatric history.

[advice on page 46]

STATION 5

Mrs Robson is a 55-year-old housewife. She attended outpatients reluctantly, reporting continuous apprehension, tension all over and an inability to relax at any point during the day. You see her and learn that she has had these symptoms for 5 months. On examination, she is fidgety, flushed, sweaty and tachycardic and appears anxious. She has never used illicit substances and she does not drink alcohol

Her GP is on the phone. He has been concerned about Mrs Robson and wants to know your differential diagnosis.

[advice on page 48]

STATION 6

A young man is brought to your clinic by his brother. The brother has become increasingly concerned about the young man's 'odd behaviour' – in particular, ideas that his family are attempting to take away his thoughts by using a computer. There have also been reports of difficulties at the garage where he works as an apprentice mechanic. He does not drink alcohol or use illegal drugs. This has never happened before and he is described as a hard-working individual.

Assess his thoughts and beliefs.

[advice on page 50]

STATION 7

Assess this woman, who thinks that her eyes are spaced too widely apart.

[advice on page 52]

STATION 8

A 23-year-old carpenter presents to your outpatients' department reporting loss of interest in his work and poor sleep. He was reluctant to attend, as in his view it is nothing to do with mental health.

Examine this gentleman, eliciting any possible psychopathology.

[advice on page 54]

STATION 9

This patient complains of tremor and weakness over a number of weeks.

Perform a neurological examination of his upper limbs.

Do not use pinprick as part of your assessment.

[advice on page 56]

STATION 10

This woman has been drinking alcohol heavily for years and now suffers with oesophageal reflux. She claims that she wants to stop drinking.

Explore her attitudes, beliefs and expectations with regards to her drinking.

She wants to know about alcohol detoxification.

[advice on page 58]

STATION 11

Mr Lewis's wife has just been admitted to the ward. She has been diagnosed with depression, having tried to take an overdose. She was discovered by their son, who called for help.

Mr Lewis wants to know more about depression, in particular what causes it and whether his wife will get better.

[advice on page 61]

STATION 12

Miss Peterson is a 36-year-old unemployed woman who presents to the accident and emergency department, having cut her wrists at home. Her injuries are superficial and do not require medical intervention. She has had a few alcoholic drinks and is a little upset.

Take a history from Miss Peterson, eliciting the important features of emotionally unstable personality disorder.

[advice on page 63]

STATION 1: CLOZAPINE

THE EXAMINER'S MARK SHEET	
Communication skills	Risks/benefits
Rapport	Answering other questions
Explanation	Global rating

INTRODUCE YOURSELF

'Hello, nice to meet you. My name is Dr Smith.'

SET THE SCENE

'I've been asked by your consultant and the rest of the team looking after you to talk to you about your treatment. Would that be OK?'

'You've had a number of years now on different medications and they haven't helped as much as we had hoped.'

'We hope that a different medication will be more effective. It has worked well for many people in a similar situation to you.'

FIND OUT WHAT HE ALREADY KNOWS

'Have you heard about a medication called clozapine?'

'What do you know about it?'

INFORMATION ON CLOZAPINE TREATMENT

Sometimes, the actor is instructed to fire questions at you before you have a chance to get into your stride. You will score highly if you remain calm.

'Are there any side effects?'

'Yes, as with every medication there are side effects. Some are common and some are rare. Many of these should wear off after 3–4 weeks. Possible common side effects include sedation, increased salivation, increase or decrease in blood pressure, fever and nausea.'

'It also causes weight gain, but we will help you to watch this and can give you dietary advice.'

'The most serious side effect is a drop in the white blood cells (those that fight infection), but this is rare. As a precaution, though, we need to monitor patients prescribed clozapine by taking blood samples.'

'Ideally, we like to start clozapine in hospital at first, but we could also do this from home with close monitoring.'

'It sounds awful. I'd rather not.'

'Of course, not everyone gets all of the side effects, but I think it's important to tell you about these things. What I can tell you is that it's a very effective drug and you should feel reassured, as we will be monitoring you very closely.'

'It helps many people with schizophrenia and has a low incidence of other side effects like tremor and unwanted movements, which you can get with some of the other medications.'

'No, I think I'll stay on what I'm taking already.'

'Why don't you have a think about it and we can meet again.'

'Perhaps you would like to talk to your friends or family or some patients who take clozapine and see what they have to say?'

Avoid getting into battles with patients. You will not fail because you could not persuade him, on one occasion, to take a medication, but you might fail if you become irritable with him.

ASK WHETHER HE HAS ANY OTHER QUESTIONS

THANK HIM

FOR EXTRA MARKS

Other side effects include constipation, tachycardia, seizures and nocturnal enuresis.

Other serious adverse effects include thromboembolism, cardiomyopathy and myocarditis.

Risk of developing agranulocytosis: 0.8 per cent.

Risk of developing neutropenia: 3 per cent.

Patients must be registered with a monitoring service, e.g. the Clozaril patient monitoring service (CPMS).

Blood sampling weekly for 18 weeks, then fortnightly until 52 weeks, and monthly thereafter.

Weak dopamine D1 and D2 receptor antagonist; higher affinity for dopamine D4, serotonin 5HT2 and 5HT3, and adrenergic $\alpha 1$ and $\alpha 2$ receptors.

Does not raise prolactin levels.

Care if history of seizures: risk increases significantly at or above 600 mg daily.

Cigarette-smoking reduces efficacy.

FURTHER READING

Serretti A, De Ronchi D, Lorenzi C, Berardi D. New antipsychotics and schizophrenia: a review of efficacy and side effects. *Curr Med Chem* 2004; 11: 343–58.

STATION 2: DRUG-RELATED WEIGHT GAIN

THE EXAMINER'S MARK SHEET	
Communication skills	Risks of stopping medication
Empathy	Advice on weight gain
Explanation of side effects	Global rating

INTRODUCE YOURSELF

'Hello, nice to meet you. My name is Dr Smith.'

SET THE SCENE

'I understand you have put on some weight over the past 9 months and that this seems to tie in with having started olanzapine. Is that correct?'
'I'm sorry to hear you have put on weight. Is it something that concerns you?'

FIND OUT WHAT THEY ALREADY KNOW

'What do you know about olanzapine?'
'Has anyone talked to you at any point about the side effects of this medication?'
Weight gain can cause considerable upset to patients. Where possible, information about the common and important rare side effects should always be made available to patients before starting medication.

INFORMATION ON MEDICATION

Weight gain

Olanzapine does have the potential for weight gain. It is thought to do this by increasing appetite. The exact mechanisms for this are unclear. It might help to explain that the weight gain is common with this medication and that this should have been explained to her as a potential side effect.

Stopping the medication

She has been very sensible in approaching you for advice rather than just stopping the medication. Changing the medication is preferable to stopping altogether. An atypical antipsychotic that is less likely to cause weight gain can be prescribed. It is possible that stopping may precipitate a relapse (you would need a collateral history/old notes) or worsening of symptoms.

Dietary advice

Inform her that weight gain has implications not only for self-image but also for physical health (discuss the increased risk with weight gain of diabetes and cardiovascular disease).

Dietitian input with nutritional advice is important (foods to avoid/reduce – a personalised dietary programme is helpful).

Detailed history of her diet, especially sugary drinks, fatty foods, etc., will be important.

Provide behavioural advice and education, e.g. increased exercise/exercise programme, walking rather than using transport, reduced snacking between meals.

ASK WHETHER SHE HAS ANY OTHER QUESTIONS

THANK HER

FOR EXTRA MARKS

Clozapine and olanzapine have higher potential for weight gain compared with other atypical antipsychotics.

Amisulpride and aripiprazole are less likely than other atypical antipsychotics to cause weight gain.

The exact mechanism of weight gain remains unclear. Neuroleptic interference with serotonin, histamine and prolactin activity has been suggested as a potential cause. Neuropeptides, gut hormones, adipose tissue and hair-root-derived hormones also have been implicated

FURTHER READING

Ananth J, Venkatesh R, Burgoyne K, *et al.* Atypical antipsychotic induced weight gain: pathophysiology and management. *Ann Clin Psychiatry* 2004; 16: 75–85.

STATION 3: ABDOMINAL EXAMINATION

THE EXAMINER'S MARK SHEET	
Communication/rapport	Percussion
Inspection	Auscultation
Palpation	Global rating

INTRODUCE YOURSELF

'Hello, nice to meet you. My name is Dr Smith.'

SET THE SCENE

'I have been asked to examine your stomach/tummy.'

ASK FOR PERMISSION

'Would that be OK?'

'If at any point you are uncomfortable or want me to stop, please tell me.'

'I normally have a nurse with me when I examine a patient but are you happy for me to continue?' (This lets the examiner know that you would ordinarily request a chaperone.)

CLINICAL PROCEDURE

Remember: inspection, palpation, percussion and auscultation.

Ask the patient to lie flat, with their arms by their sides.

Expose the abdomen (and chest if male).

Inspection

Look for any obvious abnormalities/clinical signs, e.g. spider naevi, gynaecomastia, tattoos, jaundice, pigmentation, abdominal distension (ascites), loss of body hair, scars, fistulae and pulsations.

Examine the hands for clubbing, palmar erythema, Dupuytren's contracture and flapping tremor.

Palpation

Feel the neck and supraclavicular fossae for enlarged lymph nodes (lymph nodes, particularly in the left supraclavicular fossa, may be enlarged in carcinoma of the stomach).

Light palpation: in all four quadrants. Look at the patient's face and ask whether there is any tenderness.

Deeper palpation: as above, and also mid-line for possible aortic aneurysm.

Examine the main organs individually:

Liver: start in right lower quadrant and work upwards.
Spleen: start in right lower quadrant and move across to left upper quadrant.
Kidneys: bilateral palpation of lateral abdomen.

Tell the examiner that ordinarily you would also examine for inguinal lymphadenopathy.

Percussion
From the level of the nipple downwards, percuss out the sizes of the liver and the spleen:

The edges of both organs should become apparent.
Shifting dullness should be demonstrated if ascites is suspected.
Abdominal fluid is stony dull on percussion.

Auscultation
Bowel sounds
Renal artery bruits

THANK THE PATIENT

FOR EXTRA MARKS

Talk through your examination as you go, so the examiner knows you are doing all the right things, e.g. 'I'm just looking at your hands for any changes in your nails. Have you noticed any changes yourself?'

Comment on any abnormalities.

Explain to the examiner that a complete abdominal examination would include examination of the male external genitalia and rectal examination, but that these would not be appropriate in all circumstances, and certainly not without a chaperone.

STATION 4: THYROID EXAMINATION

THE EXAMINER'S MARK SHEET	
Communication/rapport	Percussion
Inspection	Auscultation
Palpation	Global rating

INTRODUCE YOURSELF

'Hello, nice to meet you. My name is Dr Smith.'

SET THE SCENE

'I understand that you've noticed your neck seems to be enlarged. Lithium treatment can interfere with the thyroid gland, causing it to enlarge, so I would like to examine your neck.'

ASK FOR PERMISSION

'Would that be OK?'
'Let me know if you are uncomfortable at any point.'

CLINICAL PROCEDURE

Remember: inspection, palpation, percussion and auscultation.
The patient should be sitting.

Inspection
Expose the neck.
Make a show of looking at the thyroid from the front. A goitre or nodular thyroid should be visible.
Look at the patient's eyes from the sides and from above (exophthalmos).
Ask the subject to take some water into the mouth and to hold it there.
Again, make a show of watching any goitre move upwards as the patient swallows.

Palpation
Ask the patient for permission to feel his neck.
Stand behind him and to the right. This is less threatening than standing directly behind.
With your fingers from both hands, feel the left and right lobes of the thyroid.
Assess hard or soft texture and the presence of any nodules.
Assess the extent of any enlargement.

Again, ask the patient to swallow some water whilst feeling a possible goitre move beneath the examining fingers.

Examine local lymph nodes, as thyroid carcinoma can spread to local lymphatics.

Percussion

Percuss the manubrium sterni to see whether a goitre extends downwards (dullness) into the chest.

Auscultation

If a stethoscope is available, listen to both lobes of the thyroid for bruits and then the chest for arrhythmias.

THANK THE PATIENT

FOR EXTRA MARKS

Examine the hands for tremor (hyperthyroidism).

Examine the eyes for exophthalmos/proptosis (Graves' disease), lid retraction and lid lag.

Auscultate for cardiac arrhythmias (tachycardia, atrial fibrillation, bradycardia).

Comment on the patient's weight (gain/loss).

Comment on any hair loss, dry flaky skin, lateral loss of eyebrows, hoarse croaky voice and carpel tunnel syndrome (hypothyroidism).

Examine for brisk/slowed tendon reflexes (hyper/hypothyroid, respectively).

Enquire about intolerance to heat/cold.

Ask about increased agitation (hyperthyroid).

STATION 5: GENERALISED ANXIETY DISORDER

THE EXAMINER'S MARK SHEET	
Communication skills	Management
Preferred diagnosis	Answering other questions
Differential diagnosis	Global rating

Much here depends on what the GP says, but the same principles apply. Remember to avoid lay terms in this station.

INTRODUCE YOURSELF

'Hello, it's Dr Smith here. May I ask who I'm talking to?'

SET THE SCENE

'I've seen Mrs Robson. I understand you would like to know her differential diagnosis. Is this correct?'

FIND OUT WHAT THEY ALREADY KNOW

'Do you know whether Mrs Robson has ever been diagnosed with mental illness before or whether this is her first presentation?'
'Is she prescribed any medication?'
'Has anything in her life/circumstances changed recently that you know about?
'From my meeting with her today, it seems that the most likely diagnosis is an anxiety disorder. Do you know much about anxiety disorders?'

INFORMATION ON ANXIETY

Most likely diagnosis

Generalised anxiety disorder (GAD) – if anxiety is 'free-floating' (pervasive and unfocused).

Differential diagnosis

Other anxiety disorders, e.g. social phobia, agoraphobia, panic disorder, PTSD
Medical disorder, e.g. hyperthyroidism (common), phaeochromocytoma
Affective disorder
Psychotic disorder

Management
Medication
SSRIs, venlafaxine (SNRI).

Benzodiazepines can be useful in the first 2 weeks as a short-term measure (emergency treatment) – but controversial approach, addictive potential.

Some tricyclic antidepressants are useful.

Psychotherapy
Cognitive-behavioural therapy and self-help techniques give better results than placebo over a 10-week period (*Lancet* 1988; **30**: 235–40).

ASK WHETHER THE GP HAS ANY OTHER QUESTIONS

THANK HIM

FOR EXTRA MARKS

Anxiety-management techniques have been shown to be useful. Booklets explaining the origins of anxiety symptoms, relaxation exercises, distraction techniques, control of unwanted thoughts and techniques to raise self-confidence can be helpful.

In primary-care and non-psychiatric populations, cognitive therapy has been shown to be effective in maintaining gains over 3 months.

Of all the anxiety disorders, GAD has the highest comorbidity rates.

FURTHER READING

Tonks A. Treating generalised anxiety disorder. *Br Med J* 2003; **326**: 700–702.

STATION 6: PSYCHOSIS

THE EXAMINER'S MARK SHEET	
Communication skills	Risk considered
Thought passivity	Answering other questions
Thought content	Global rating

INTRODUCE YOURSELF

'Hello, nice to meet you. My name is Dr Smith.'

SET THE SCENE

Remember to use open questions to start. This allows the patient to explain in their own words:
'Your brother brought you here today to see me. Do you know why?'
'I wanted to ask you whether anything has been troubling you recently?'
'I wondered whether you felt things have been happening to you that you find hard to explain?'

ASK FOR PERMISSION

'Can we talk about that?'

TAKE A HISTORY OF THOUGHTS AND BELIEFS: KEY AREAS

Really you are assessing thought content and any preoccupations. From the history, you will be interested in thought passivity/possession and delusions/overvalued ideas. Abnormalities in the form of thought will become apparent from the patient's use of language.

Thought possession

Use open questions to start.

Thought insertion: 'Are you able to think clearly or is anything interfering with your thoughts?'
'Are thoughts put into your head that are not your own?'
Thought broadcast: 'Do you hear your own thoughts spoken aloud so that people standing near to you could hear them too?'
Thought echo/running commentary: 'Do you ever hear your own thoughts echoed or repeated?'
Thought withdrawal: 'Are your own thoughts ever removed from your head as though someone or something was taking them out?'
Thought stopping: 'Do your thoughts ever stop suddenly and unexpectedly, when your thinking was fine moments before?'

Thought content, delusions

Use open questions to start: 'Sometimes I see people who have had unusual things happening to them. Has anything like this happened to you?' (normalising).

The patient says: 'What do you mean?'

Delusions of control: 'For example, some people feel that they are under the control of some force or power other than themselves. Has this been happening to you?'

Delusions of reference: 'Do people drop hints about you or say things with a double meaning?'

Delusional misinterpretation/misidentification: 'Do things seem to be specially arranged?'

Delusions of persecution: 'Is anyone or anything trying to hurt or harm you in away?'

Delusional perception: 'Has anything happened recently that has been very meaningful or of great significance to you?' (e.g. 'A traffic light changed to red and I knew I had been chosen to lead my people.')

Remember *risk*: ask whether he is having thoughts about harming himself or others.

ASK WHETHER THEY HAVE ANY QUESTIONS

THANK THEM

FOR EXTRA MARKS

It is important to differentiate delusions from overvalued ideas if you identify unusual beliefs.

Time permitting, you should also ask about delusional explanations for any unusual or paranormal phenomena.

Other possible delusions: grandiose abilities/identity, religious ideas, jealousy, guilt, nihilism, appearance.

FURTHER READING

Sims A. *Symptoms in the Mind: An Introduction to Descriptive Psychopathology.* London: Balliere Tindall, 2002.

STATION 7: BODY DYSMORPHIC DISORDER

THE EXAMINER'S MARK SHEET	
Communication skills	Delusion/overvalued idea
Empathy	Answering other questions
History of complaint	Global rating

INTRODUCE YOURSELF

'Hello, nice to meet you. My name is Dr Smith.'

SET THE SCENE

'I've been told that you have some concerns about your appearance. Is that correct?'
'Can we talk about this?'

ASK FOR PERMISSION

'Is that OK?'

ASSESSMENT OF BODY DYSMORPHIC DISORDER: KEY AREAS

Interestingly, this is an exam favourite. However, the Part I OSCE is testing basic skills, not an in-depth knowledge of body dysmorphic disorder (BDD). Therefore, what is being examined at this station is the ability to test a delusional system.

Basic history

Try to get some information around the perceived defect, e.g. what this involves, when it started and any steps taken to change the supposed abnormality, e.g. surgery. Has the problem led to preoccupation, ruminating, checking in mirrors and seeking reassurance?
Have there been any concerns about other body parts in the past?

Elicit BDD psychopathology

A little knowledge about BDD is necessary. This is a clinical condition in which there is a preoccupation with a defect that is imaginary and generally not present. If a minor defect is present, then it is significantly less than that which the patient perceives. As in this case, the defect often features some part of the head. Other common preoccupations are with a perceived big nose, protruding ears and an abnormal hairline.
BDD may present in the form of an overvalued idea, a hypochondriacal disorder

or a delusional disorder, in which the belief system is unshakeable. Test whether the belief expressed *is delusional, or not.*

BDD also can be part of another disorder, e.g. a greater delusional disorder, OCD, social phobia or major depressive disorder.

Generally, there is low self-esteem and patients consider themselves unattractive and ugly.

ASK WHETHER SHE HAS ANY QUESTIONS

THANK HER

FOR EXTRA MARKS

Explore the patient's ideas surrounding the perceived abnormality:

Patient: 'My eyes are spaced too widely apart.'

Candidate: 'I didn't notice that. Do you worry about this? Has this always been the case? Have you always thought this?'

Patient:

(1)

– Yes, I have.
– I don't think it: I *know* it.
– Always, since I was a kid.

or

(2)

– Yeah, sometimes it bothers me more than other times.
– I know it is a bit silly but I can't help it.

Candidate: For response (1) above, you have to test the delusionary system: Could there be any other explanation for the situation? For instance, 'I have seen people in the past reporting abnormalities that were not as bad as they thought ... in some instances, they were not there at all. Could this possibly be happening in your case?'

If the answer is 'no', then the diagnosis is most probably delusional BDD. If insight is present and the answer is 'maybe', then the diagnosis is most likely an overvalued idea.

Delusional disorder and non-delusional-based BDD show little difference when compared in terms of demographics, phenomenology, course, associated features and treatment response (*Psychopharmacol Bull* 1994; **30**: 179–86); both respond to SSRIs (*J Clin Psychiatry* 1993; **54**: 389–95).

FURTHER READING

McElroy SL, Phillips KA, Keck PE, Hudson JI, Pope HG. Body dysmorphic disorder: does it have a psychotic subtype? *J Clin Psychiatry* 1993; **54**: 389–95.

Phillips KA, McElroy SL, Keck PE, Hudson JI, Pope HG. A comparison of delusional and non delusional body dysmorphic disorder in 100 cases. *Psychopharmacol Bull* 1994; **30**: 179–86.

STATION 8: FEATURES OF DEPRESSION

THE EXAMINER'S MARK SHEET	
Communication skills	Suicidality/homicidality
Core depressive features	Biological/somatic features
Associated features	Global rating

INTRODUCE YOURSELF

'Hello, nice to meet you. My name is Dr Smith.'

SET THE SCENE

Always start with a warm and engaging introduction:
'Many thanks for attending today. I wanted to talk to you about how you've been feeling recently.'

ASK FOR PERMISSION

'Would that be OK?'

TAKE A HISTORY OF DEPRESSION: KEY AREAS

Don't forget that good candidates can be tripped up in exams by not knowing the very basics of general psychiatry. This station is a classic example. It is important to know the core features of depression – depressed *mood*, increased *fatiguability* and loss of *interest* (*MFI*).

The two symptoms offered in the example are suggestive of depression, but note also the probable lack of insight and possible hostility. It may be useful to start with the somatic features of depression, as the patient does not believe he has a mental illness.

Somatic symptoms

Insomnia or hypersomnia
Early-morning wakening
Diurnal variation in mood
Psychomotor agitation or excitation
Diminished appetite
Weight loss
Marked loss of libido

Mood

'How have you been feeling in yourself over the past few weeks?'
'Can you tell me how you've been feeling in terms of your mood?'
'Can you tell me a little more about that?'

It is important to follow through fully on examination of mood. If a response of 'a little low in mood' is offered, you must proceed to ask about thoughts of self-harm. It is essential to ask about suicide at this station.

'Sometimes, when people feel low, thoughts about harming themselves can creep in. Have you had any of these thoughts? That must be very difficult ... did these thoughts ever get to the point where you wished you were dead? Do you still feel like that now?'

Other common features

Diminished interest or pleasure
Poor self-esteem and loss of confidence
Feelings of worthlessness and guilt
Recurrent thoughts of death or self-harm
Hopelessness with regard to the future
Poor concentration and attention

Psychosis

Delusions and hallucinations may also be present (severe depressive episode) and so should be enquired about.

ASK WHETHER HE HAS ANY QUESTIONS

THANK HIM

FOR EXTRA MARKS

The extra marks at this station will go for sensitivity around any possible hostility that the man holds for attending a psychiatrist.

If this is a hostile patient, then launching in with questions will only serve to irritate the patient further. Hostility, irritability and aggressiveness, although not typical, can be presenting features of depression.

SUPPORT GROUPS/ADVICE

Depression Alliance: www.depressionalliance.org

FURTHER READING

Learn the features of depression from ICD-10.

STATION 9: UPPER-LIMB EXAMINATION

THE EXAMINER'S MARK SHEET	
Communication skills	Reflexes
Inspection/positioning	Sensation
Tone/power	Global rating

INTRODUCE YOURSELF

'Hello, nice to meet you. My name is Dr Smith.'

SET THE SCENE

'I've been told you've had some shaking and weakness in your arms and hands. Is that right? I'd like to examine you.'

ASK FOR PERMISSION

'Would that be OK?'
'Let me know if you are uncomfortable at any point.'

CLINICAL PROCEDURE

The patient should, ideally, be on an examination couch.
Examine from the patient's right-hand side.

By explaining what you are doing at each step, you are letting the examiner know that you are competent.

Inspection

Look for: Any obvious abnormalities/deformities in the arms and hands
Skin colour/rashes
Muscle wasting
Muscle fasciculation (motor neurone disease)
Tremor (EPSE, Parkinson's disease)

Tone

Examine each arm by moving it passively at the elbow joint to and fro. Flex and extend the hand at the wrist and rotate the hand. This should detect cogwheel or lead-pipe rigidity.

Power

Ask the subject to:

Put arms at right-angles to their body: 'Don't let me push them down.'
Bend elbow: 'Don't let me straighten it.'

Push out straight each arm against your resistance.
'Squeeze my fingers': offer two fingers.
Keep fingers straight: 'Don't let me bend them.'
Spread out their fingers: 'Don't let me push them together.'
Point your thumb to the ceiling: 'Don't let me push it down.'
Put their thumb and little finger together: 'Don't let me pull them apart.'

Co-ordination

'Tap quickly on the back of your hand.'
'Touch my finger – touch your nose' test.

Reflexes

Biceps jerk (C5, C6)
Triceps jerk (C7)
Supinator (C5, C6)

Sensation

Ideally, one should test light touch (cotton-wool) and pinprick (not here) in the following areas (although, for the purposes of the exam, a finger touch should suffice):

Shoulder (C4, C5)
Upper arm (C5, C6)
Forearm (C6, C7, T1)
Hand (C6, C7, C8)

Ask the subject to close their eyes and tell you when they feel something. Reassure them that you will be gentle. Compare right hand with left hand, etc.

THANK THE PATIENT

FOR EXTRA MARKS

Vibration sense and joint position also can be tested.
Comment on any abnormalities as you find them.
Knowing the nerve routes may earn you extra marks but is probably not necessary to pass.

STATION 10: ALCOHOL MISUSE AND OESOPHAGEAL REFLUX

THE EXAMINER'S MARK SHEET	
Communication/rapport	Alcohol detoxification explanation
Attitude to alcohol	Answering other questions
Beliefs and expectations	Global rating

INTRODUCE YOURSELF

'Hello, nice to meet you. My name is Dr Smith.'

SET THE SCENE

'I'm sorry to hear that you've been troubled by reflux. I know this can be very uncomfortable.'

'I would like to learn more about your alcohol intake and how you feel about this.'

ASK FOR PERMISSION

'Would that be OK?'

TAKE A HISTORY OF ALCOHOL MISUSE AND ATTITUDES TO DRINKING: KEY AREAS

Current habits

First, find out from the patient what 'drinking heavily' means. If it is indeed heavy alcohol use, then is she dependent?

A very rough but sometimes useful questionnaire is the *CAGE*:

Do you feel you should *cut* down on your drinking?
Do you get *annoyed* when you are criticised regarding your drinking?
Do you feel *guilty* about your drinking?
Do you have an *eye-opener* in the morning?
More than two positive responses is thought to indicate problem drinking.

Attitudes, beliefs and expectations

A key issue with treatment and any type of change in addiction is *motivation*. Exploring the woman's attitudes allows an assessment of her reasons for continuing to drink and whether she is in a position to change.

A useful technique used in motivational interviewing is drawing up a *balance sheet* with the patient of the positive and negative issues of continuing to drink. Do this quickly in one statement:

'Sometimes it is useful to have a look at the benefits of continuing or stopping alcohol. Can you come up with a few positives and negatives?'

Attitudes and beliefs will quickly become apparent when drawing up a balance sheet.

It would be useful to draw attention to the oesophageal reflux as a result of alcohol use. The patient should be aware that heavy alcohol may have led to this.

Alcohol detoxification

Try to establish whether she is interested in getting help first:

Has she had any treatments before?
What did that involve?

'I understand that you are interested in alcohol detoxification. We can do this either in the community or as an inpatient.'

The preferred method is as an inpatient, because withdrawal phenomena can be monitored. If any physical complications, such as seizures, arise, they can be treated more effectively in the inpatient setting. Also, if high-level benzodiazepines have to be prescribed, then an initial 48-hour assessment can be performed and the side effects of the medication monitored closely.

After the acute phase, a period of rehabilitation is sometimes appropriate. This is very much dependent on the severity of the person's drinking and their social circumstances, e.g. family and work. This can be for a period of up to 6 months or even longer. The rehabilitation unit provides an environment of individual and group sessions to strengthen coping mechanisms in dealing with alcohol. All the time, this is conducted in a drug- and alcohol-free environment.

ASK WHETHER SHE HAS ANY QUESTIONS

THANK HER

FOR EXTRA MARKS

It is important to establish whether the patient views the alcohol intake as harmful. Advanced alcoholism can be accompanied by partial or complete lack of insight.

Good prognostic factors: motivated
insightful
good support (family/friends).

Benzodiazepines are drugs of choice for alcohol withdrawal.
Parenteral supplements (e.g. Pabrinex®) are important to prevent/treat Wernicke–Korsakoff syndrome.

SUPPORT GROUPS/ADVICE

Alcoholics Anonymous: www.alcoholics-anonymous.org.uk

FURTHER READING

Claassen CA, Adinoff B. Alcohol withdrawal syndrome: guidelines for management. *CNS Drugs* 1999; 12: 279–91.

STATION 11: DEPRESSION

THE EXAMINER'S MARK SHEET	
Communication/empathy	Prognosis
Depression explanation	Answering other questions
Aetiology	Global rating

INTRODUCE YOURSELF

'Hello, nice to meet you. My name is Dr Smith.'

SET THE SCENE

'I understand that your wife has been diagnosed with depression. You must be worried about her.'
'You wanted to find out some more about this condition. Is that correct?'

FIND OUT WHAT THEY ALREADY KNOW

'What do you already know about depression?'

INFORMATION ON DEPRESSION

'We all experience low mood now and then, but the feelings involved in clinical depression are much stronger, more unpleasant and more persistent. These symptoms often last for months and sometimes longer still. You may have noticed that your wife has lost interest in things and is easily tired, in addition to having low mood. These are typical findings in depression.'
'Have you noticed any other symptoms?'
(Refer to Exam 2, Station 8 for other depressive symptoms.)
In reference to the overdose: 'Sometimes things can seem so desperate that they feel that life is no longer worth living.'

Aetiology

'The cause for depression is not always clear. Sometimes it can follow a stressful life event, but for some people it is less obvious.'

Genetic factors: 'A family history of depression increases your risk of becoming depressed yourself. If you have one parent with depression, then you are around eight times more likely to develop depression.'

Personality: 'Certain types of personality might mean you are more likely to become depressed' (e.g. dysthymic personality).

Precipitating factors: 'Stressful life events, such as losing one's job, may cause a depressive episode.'

Predisposing factors: 'Adverse life events occurring in childhood or ongoing difficulties, for example at work or at home, can also lead to depression.'

Physical illness: 'Some medical (usually chronic) disorders have a strong association with depression, e.g. glandular fever, Parkinson's disease and cardiovascular disease.'

Gender: 'Although anyone can become depressed, women are at greater risk than men.'

Prognosis

Individual episodes: prognosis very good (although recurrence is common). However, 50–75 per cent relapse, and 25–30 per cent become chronic.

'With treatment, each episode lasts 2–3 months on average, but a minority last for much longer (years).'

ASK HIM WHETHER HE HAS ANY QUESTIONS

THANK HIM

FOR EXTRA MARKS

It is recommended that antidepressants are continued for a least a year after recovery.
Psychotherapy (CBT) helps patients to counter automatic negative thoughts.

SUPPORT GROUPS/ADVICE

Depression Alliance: www.depressionalliance.org
Fellowship of Depressives Anonymous:
www.zenforge.pwp.blueyonder.co.uk/fda/
Relate: www.relate.org.uk
Samaritans: www.samaritans.org.uk/
Hospital users'/patients' groups

FURTHER READING

Mynors-Wallis LM, Gath DH, Day A, Baker F. Randomised controlled trial of problem-solving treatment, antidepressant medication, and combined treatment for major depression in primary care. *Br Med J* 2000; **320**: 26–30.

STATION 12: EMOTIONALLY UNSTABLE PERSONALITY DISORDER

THE EXAMINER'S MARK SHEET	
Communication/rapport	Current suicidal risk
History of this episode	Answering other questions
Features of emotionally unstable personality disorder	Global rating

INTRODUCE YOURSELF

'Hello, nice to meet you. My name is Dr Smith.'

SET THE SCENE

'I'm sorry to hear you've injured your wrists.'
'Could we talk about what happened?'

ASK FOR PERMISSION

'Would that be OK?'

TAKE A HISTORY OF EMOTIONALLY UNSTABLE PERSONALITY DISORDER: KEY AREAS

An empathetic response, but with firm boundaries, is important.
Allow time for silence and for the patient to speak.

Brief history

What precipitated this episode?
Was the intent to die or to self-harm (final acts, methods to avoid discovery)?
Current suicidal intent (very important)?
How did she get to the A&E department?
Previous episodes of self-harm?

You must elicit at least some of the following features:

Emotionally unstable personality disorder (PD) (impulsive type)

Unstable mood:	'Do you find your mood changes from day to day or from week to week?'
Desultory (superficial):	'Do your goals in life tend to change depending, for instance, on how you are feeling?'
Explosivity:	'We all become upset from time to time. Do certain people upset you from time to time? What usually happens when you become upset?'

| Quarrelsome: | 'We all have arguments, but do you find you have many arguments?' |
| Unpredictability: | 'Do you ever lose control in certain situations and perhaps become upset or even aggressive?' |

Emotionally unstable PD (borderline type)

Unstable mood and emotions.

Self-harm:	'Did you harm yourself today because certain thoughts and feelings became too much to deal with? Have you ever harmed yourself in the past?'
Relationship difficulties/crises:	'Have you had any relationship difficulties recently or in the past?'
Feelings of emptiness:	'Do you ever feel low and empty inside from time to time?'
Poor self-image:	'How do you feel about yourself most of the time?'

ASK WHETHER SHE HAS ANY QUESTIONS

THANK HER

FOR EXTRA MARKS

Borderline PD affects one to two per cent of the population.
Male : Female 1 : 2.

FURTHER READING

Casey PR, Tyrer P. Personality disorder and psychiatric illness in general practice. *Br J Psychiatry* 1990; **156**: 261–5.

EXAM 3

STATION 1

This 28-year-old secretary began hearing voices 2 months ago. She was seen by her local community psychiatric services and diagnosed with schizophrenia. Her consultant psychiatrist has limited experience with the newer antipsychotics and prefers prescribing the older traditional drugs. She was given 100 mg chlorpromazine daily but she stopped taking it altogether after complaining of uncomfortable legs, stiffness and a feeling of 'unease'. Her community psychiatric nurse is concerned that she is refusing further treatment and has asked you to see her.

Assess this patient for extrapyramidal side effects.
Explain to the patient what you believe has happened.
What other treatment options are available?

[advice on page 70]

STATION 2

This 72-year-old retired solicitor has noticed that his memory is deteriorating. He frequently forgets where he has placed things. His wife is concerned as he recently lost £300 in cash and she has had to take over running the finances at home. He is finding it increasingly difficult to remember appointments and has been leaving notes for himself everywhere as prompts. His wife feels that he is becoming increasingly stubborn and querulous. He has stopped watercolour-painting, which used to be his favourite hobby.

He has a medical history of hypertension, for which he is prescribed bendroflumethiazide (bendrofluazide). Clinical examination is unremarkable, including CNS. He has no past psychiatric history.

Carry out a cognitive assessment.

[advice on page 73]

STATION 3

Mrs Smith, a 35-year-old accountant, has been suffering panic attacks with increased frequency. She has been told that the condition she is suffering from is panic disorder.

She does not understand why this is happening to her, and she asks you to explain the cause of panic attacks.

Explain to her how panic attacks occur.

[advice on page 76]

STATION 4

Mr Andrews is a 36-year-old painter and decorator. He suffered a severe beating by a group of youths on a bus while travelling home from work late one evening. Although he has never had problems in the past, he now describes persistent anxiety and difficulty in sleeping at night.

Take a history from Mr Andrews, eliciting the key features of his difficulties.

[advice on page 78]

STATION 5

Mr Shah is a 39-year-old teacher from the local area who has recently been suspended from work having been discovered drunk at school on two occasions. His family doctor has informed him that he is alcohol-dependent and has referred him to you at the addiction clinic for assessment and further treatment. He attends with his wife, who is very supportive but concerned as he has been increasingly aggressive of late.

Take an alcohol history.

[advice on page 80]

STATION 6

This depressed patient has failed to respond to three separate therapeutic courses of antidepressant medication. Your consultant thinks he should have a course of electroconvulsive therapy (ECT).

Give him information about ECT.

He asks about the effect on his memory.

[advice on page 82]

STATION 7

An elderly woman has become increasingly concerned that her neighbours are attempting to poison her with gas. She has been shouting at people outside her home. She is clearly upset, and the police have been called. They persuade her to come to hospital. She has been seen by a psychiatric liaison nurse, who has asked you to assess her. The nurse informs you that the woman is 77 years old, lives alone and has no next of kin. The nurse has contacted the general practitioner, and there is no past history of mental illness.

Assess her for formal thought disorder and abnormal perceptions.

[advice on page 85]

STATION 8

This nurse has asked for your opinion about a 35-year-old patient who has become increasingly unwell over the past 12 hours. His GP has seen him and could not find a physical cause after examining him and excluding an infection. He has been feeling nauseous, sweaty and agitated. He is being treated for mixed anxiety and depression with paroxetine, the dose of which was increased yesterday.

Explain to the nurse what you think is the most likely diagnosis.
Tell the nurse the features of your preferred diagnosis.
The nurse wants to know what the plan is.

[advice on page 87]

STATION 9

This is the 42-year-old daughter of a woman recently diagnosed with Alzheimer's disease, at the age of 65 years. The daughter is not certain what this diagnosis means and had thought that her mother's worsening memory was just part of getting older. She is now extremely concerned, not only about her mother's future but also about the risk to herself and her own children.

Explain to the daughter what a diagnosis of dementia means and its prognosis.
Discuss the risk that she herself will develop Alzheimer's disease.
She wants to know whether she and her children should have genetic testing and whether taking supplements like ginkgo biloba will help reduce their risks.

[advice on page 90]

STATION 10

Mr Cohen's son has just been diagnosed with bipolar affective disorder. He has been an inpatient in a psychiatric ward for the past 2 months.

Mr Cohen wants to speak to you about bipolar disorder and is looking for advice.

[advice on page 92]

STATION 11

A 31-year-old antiques dealer was admitted to your ward some time ago with a florid psychosis. Your team has confirmed a diagnosis of paranoid schizophrenia.

You have been asked to break the news to the patient.

[advice on page 94]

STATION 12

You are the psychiatrist responsible for inpatients on a detoxification ward.

A 37-year-old gentleman has been admitted for alcohol detoxification. He has very little insight into the fact that he is alcohol-dependent. He appears to believe that there is little harm in drinking, as his father and mother drank all the time and it never affected them.

Speak to this man, explaining the hazards of continuing to drink alcohol.

[advice on page 96]

STATION 1: EXTRAPYRAMIDAL SIDE EFFECTS

THE EXAMINER'S MARK SHEET	
Communication	Explanation
Empathy	Treatment options
Examination of EPSE	Global rating

INTRODUCE YOURSELF

'Hello, my name's Dr Smith. I'm sorry to hear you have had some problems with the medication.'
Reassure the patient and sympathise with her.

SET THE SCENE

'I wanted to examine you for some of the side effects you've been experiencing.'

ASK FOR PERMISSION

'Would that be OK?'
Tell her that you usually have a female chaperone present, but ask whether in these circumstances she would be happy for you to continue.

CLINICAL PROCEDURE

The patient should be sitting in a chair.
Tell the patient to inform you if she is uncomfortable at any point.
Talk through your examination so the examiner knows what you are doing.

This examination is based on the Simpson–Angus scale and the Abnormal Involuntary Movement Scale.

Global

Observe for restlessness, inability to sit/stand still and anxiety/tenseness.

Face

Expression:	observe movements of the forehead, eyebrows, peri-orbital area, cheeks, frowning, blinking, smiling or grimacing.
Lips/peri-oral:	puckering, pouting, lip-smacking.
Jaw:	biting, clenching, lateral movements.
Tongue:	increased movement in and out.
Salivation:	look under the tongue for increased/pooling of saliva.
Glabellar tap:	tap forehead gently with index finger. Parkinsonian patients continue to blink instead of accommodating after several taps.

Upper limbs

Inspect for abnormal resting movements, e.g. choreic/athetoid movements.

Arm *dropping:*   Ask the patient to stand, put out her arms and then let the arms drop.
Demonstrate for the patient.
In unaffected individuals, the arms fall freely with a slap and rebound.

Elbow rigidity: Place one hand on the forearm and the other at the elbow. Move back and forth. Feel for stiffness and resistance (lead-pipe and cogwheel rigidity).

Wrist rigidity: as above, except examine flexion, extension, lateral, medial and rotational movements.

Lower limbs

Legs: Observe the resting legs, e.g. for restlessness.
If possible, examine the patient on a bench so that the feet do not touch the ground.
Ask the patient to swing their legs (demonstrate if necessary).
Look to see whether legs swing freely or there is resistance.

Gait: Ask the patient to walk five to ten paces away and then back again. Is there reduced arm swing, stiff gait or a stooped shuffling gait?

EXPLAIN WHAT HAS HAPPENED

Inform the patient that her symptoms are very likely to be a side effect of the medication, which can happen sometimes. Acknowledge that this can feel very unpleasant. The medication she has been taking is known to act on a certain dopamine receptor (D2) that is also involved in the control of movements. Thank her for telling the nurse, because we can do something about it. Newer medications have much less activity against this receptor and so are less likely to produce this effect. Arrange for the nurse to follow her up closely over the next few weeks and arrange to see the patient again in the outpatients' department. Treatment depends upon the clinical diagnosis. The patient is likely to want to discuss basic treatment options with you:

Akathisia: Reduce antipsychotic or switch to an atypical antipsychotic. Try an antimuscarinic drug, e.g. benzatropine (benztropine). Seek senior advice if there is no improvement.

Tardive dyskinesia: Think of risk factors, e.g. female, elderly. Withdraw any antimuscarinic medication. Consider withdrawing the antipsychotic or changing to an atypical antipsychotic.

THANK THE PATIENT

FOR EXTRA MARKS

Ask the patient how she feels about what has happened.

Akathisia is associated with agitation and increased risk of self-harm/suicide.

Ask whether she has had any problems swallowing (dysphagia).

If the patient is akathisic, other treatment options might include propranolol, benzodiazepines, cyproheptadine or clonidine.

If there is tardive dyskinesia, consider vitamin E, clonazepam or propranolol.

Always seek advice from a senior colleague if you are unsure. This is what would normally happen.

FURTHER READING

Gervin M, Barnes TRE. Assessment of drug-related movement disorders in schizophrenia. *Adv Psychiatr Treat* 2000; **6**: 332–4.

STATION 2: COGNITIVE ASSESSMENT

THE EXAMINER'S MARK SHEET	
Communication/rapport	Performance feedback
Empathy	Answering other questions
Cognitive assessment	Global rating

INTRODUCE YOURSELF

'Hello, nice to meet you. My name is Dr Smith.'

SET THE SCENE

'I would like to test your memory.'

ASK FOR PERMISSION

'Would that be OK?'
'Some of the things I'm going to ask you will be quite straightforward, but others will be difficult, so try not to worry if you make a few mistakes.'

CLINICAL PROCEDURE

It is advisable to memorise the MMSE. This is what we use in day-to-day practice, after all. It can be performed readily in less than 5 minutes.

			Score (30)
Orientation	What is the ...?	Year	1
		Season	1
		Month	1
		Date	1
		Day of the week	1
	Where are we?	Country	1
		County	1
		Town/village	1
		Hospital/street	1
		Ward/house number	1
Registration	Name three objects (car, ball, man)		3
Attention	Spell 'world' backwards		5
Recall	Ask for the three objects learned in registration		3
Language	Point to a pencil and a watch and ask the patient to name them		2
Repeating	Repeat: 'No ifs, ands or buts'		1
3-stage command	'Take this piece of paper in your right hand, fold it in half, and put it on the floor'		3
Reading	Please read this and do as it says. Write down on a piece of paper: 'Please close your eyes'		1
Writing	Please write a sentence of your choice (it must make sense and be grammatically correct)		1
Copying	Copy this design (angles, number of lines and overlap must be correct to score)		1

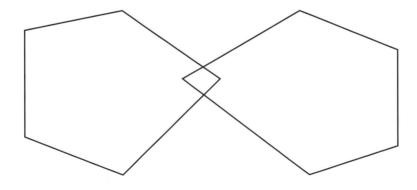

Total score____

THANK THE PATIENT

FOR EXTRA MARKS

It looks good if you can produce a MMSE score ($\leq$ 24 means probable dementia).

Give some feedback to the patient. Be realistic but encouraging.

If asked by the examiner to comment on the patient's performance, describe the areas they performed poorly in.

If appropriate and time allows, be able to test frontal, temporal and parietal lobes.

FURTHER READING

Folstein MF, Folstein SE, McHugh PR. 'Mini-mental state': a practical method for grading the cognitive state of patients for the clinician. *J Psychiatr Res* 1975; 12: 189.

STATION 3: EXPLANATION OF PANIC

THE EXAMINER'S MARK SHEET	
Communication/rapport	Psychological explanation
Empathy	Answering other questions
Aetiology	Global rating

INTRODUCE YOURSELF

'Hello, nice to meet you. My name is Dr Smith.'

SET THE SCENE

'I've been told you've been having panic attacks. Is this correct? And you wanted to find out more about panic disorder?'

FIND OUT WHAT SHE ALREADY KNOWS

'Would it be OK to ask you what you already know about panic attacks?'

INFORMATION ON PANIC

How the attacks occur

'In certain situations where we are not comfortable, such as being in crowds or feeling claustrophobic, we can become anxious. This can cause one's breathing to become shallower and faster. This change in breathing can alter the levels of certain chemicals in the body. In this case, breathing faster means the level of carbon dioxide decreases, causing particular parts of the brain to trigger more and more rapid breathing.'

'Also, depending on the individual, some people are more likely to respond to feelings of anxiety in a panicky way. An example of this would be when the chest tightens up with normal anxiety and the heart begins to beat faster; this can be perceived by some people that they are gravely ill and going to die.'

'The person never dies or suffers ill effects in the case of panic disorder.'

In panic disorder, the panic attacks occur where there is no objective danger and in unpredictable situations. The individual is usually relatively free from anxiety between attacks.

Symptoms

Palpitations
Chest pain
Choking
Dizziness   ⟹   These lead to a fear of dying
Perspiration
Depersonalisation/derealisation

Aetiology

Genetic:	increased risk among relatives of panic disorder patients (15–30 per cent).
Biochemical theory:	based on the fact that certain chemicals, e.g. sodium lactate, can induce panic attacks.
Hyperventilation theory:	overbreathing can induce panic attacks (as described above).
Cognitive model:	the patient misinterprets physical sensations such as heart palpitations as a medical emergency, e.g. a myocardial infarction. This leads to further anxiety and more physical symptoms.

ASK WHETHER SHE HAS ANY OTHER QUESTIONS

THANK HER

FOR EXTRA MARKS

If time allows, try to add in a supportive statement about the efficacy of psychological treatment.

Many individuals are helped by learning breathing exercises and controlling the hyperventilation.

Psychological therapies such as CBT help panic disorder sufferers to recognise the bodily feelings of anxiety such as shortness of breath and to relax rather than engage in hyperventilation.

Panic disorder is more common in females than in males.

FURTHER READING

Klein DF. False suffocation alarms, spontaneous panics, and related conditions: an integrative hypothesis. *Arch Gen Psychiatry* 1993; 50: 306–17.

STATION 4: POST-TRAUMATIC STRESS DISORDER

THE EXAMINER'S MARK SHEET

Communication/rapport	Comorbidity (depression/substance misuse)
Empathy	Answering other questions
Features of PTSD	Global rating

INTRODUCE YOURSELF

'Hello, nice to meet you. My name is Dr Smith.'

SET THE SCENE

'I was sorry to hear about the assault that took place on the bus.'
'I wanted to find out how you have been feeling since then.'

ASK FOR PERMISSION

'Would that be OK?'

TAKE A HISTORY OF PTSD: KEY AREAS

The description is highly suggestive of a diagnosis of PTSD. Onset usually occurs within 6 months of the event. It is important to be aware of possible differential diagnoses. In eliciting the symptoms of PTSD, you will be ruling out these diagnoses and confirming a diagnosis of PTSD.

Repeated reliving of the trauma

'When individuals suffer an unfortunate experience like yours, they can often experience dreams or nightmares. Have you experienced this at all? Sometimes one can re-experience the event in the mind, as if reliving the trauma, like a flashback ... have you ever experienced something like this before? That must have been very distressing.'

Emotional blunting and numbness

'How have you felt in yourself? Sometimes, after a distressing event, people do not feel themselves. People can sometimes describe feeling numb or detached. Have you felt this way?'

Avoidance

'Are you having any difficulty travelling? Have you been on a bus since? What happens when you travel on a bus?'

Hyperarousal, hypervigilance

'After an event like this, it is common for people to feel on edge and uneasy. Have you had any difficulties like this?' (e.g. enhanced startle reaction).

Comorbidity

Depression and substance misuse often co-occur with PTSD.
Always consider risk and enquire about suicidal intent.

OTHER REACTIONS TO SEVERE STRESS

Adjustment disorder

A significant change or life stressor leads to a short period of emotional disturbance.
Typical stressors are bereavement, divorce and new occupation.
Lasts a few days to weeks but rarely for more than 6 months.

Acute stress disorder

Time frame between PTSD and acute stress disorder is different.
With PTSD, there is supposed to be a 1-month gap before symptoms emerge, whereas with acute stress disorder, symptoms emerge immediately.

ASK WHETHER HE HAS ANY QUESTIONS

THANK HIM

FOR EXTRA MARKS

As in all OSCEs, the language you use to deliver the questions is of great importance. Practising the delivery of these questions is important.
In reality, if someone has suffered a severe trauma, we would always support them in an empathetic fashion. Don't forget to be as empathetic as possible, despite this being an artificial situation, otherwise you may lose marks.
PTSD is a difficult condition to treat (CBT, SSRIs, eye-movement desensitisation and reprocessing).
The stressor according to ICD-10 and DSM-IV typically has to be exceptionally threatening or catastrophic in nature and likely to cause distress in anyone. However, it is increasingly accepted that PTSD can be present when the stressor is less severe.

FURTHER READING

Davidson JR. Surviving disaster: what comes after the trauma? *Br J Psychiatry* 2002; 181: 366–8.

STATION 5: ALCOHOL HISTORY

THE EXAMINER'S MARK SHEET	
Communication/rapport	Risk
Empathy	Answering other questions
Alcohol history	Global rating

INTRODUCE YOURSELF

'Hello, my name is Dr Smith., It's nice to meet you both.'

If you find yourself faced with several actors, make sure you acknowledge them all.

SET THE SCENE

'Your GP has expressed some concerns about your alcohol consumption and has asked me to see you.'

'I wanted to start by talking to you about your pattern of drinking.'

ASK FOR PERMISSION

'Would that be OK?'

TAKE A HISTORY OF ALCOHOL MISUSE: KEY AREAS

Although this station is assessing mainly the candidate's ability to take an accurate history of the patient's alcohol misuse, the issue of risk (to self and others) is paramount and should be tackled at some point.

First drink

Age when first alcoholic drink consumed; type of drink.

Consequences at that time, e.g. truancy from school or loss of employment.

Drinking pattern

Typical drinking day (24-hour period).

When does he start drinking?

In the morning?

Initially at weekends then progressing to weekdays?

When has the amount consumed increased, and over what time period?

What is the most (units) consumed on a regular basis?

Does he experience withdrawal symptoms if he stops drinking?

Social impact

Occupational difficulties, e.g. time taken off work in the past, loss of job due to drinking.

Social impact, e.g. loss of friends, pastimes.

Forensic difficulties, e.g. charges for assault, drink-driving, issues of risk.

Health impact

Medical complications, e.g. ulcer, seizures, injuries.

Past detoxifications: successful or not, reasons for difficulties.

Use of other substances, especially hypnotics.

Psychiatric dual diagnosis: as high as 80 per cent. Always enquire about mood and suicide ideation.

Family history

History of alcohol dependence in family members?

ASK WHETHER THEY HAVE ANY QUESTIONS

THANK THEM

FOR EXTRA MARKS

To elicit all of the above will gain full marks with even the toughest of examiners, but being able to demonstrate a paternal history of alcohol dependence and features of antisocial personality will be impressive.

STATION 6: ELECTROCONVULSIVE THERAPY

THE EXAMINER'S MARK SHEET	
Communication	Electrode placement
ECT explanation	Answering other questions
Risks/benefits	Global rating

INTRODUCE YOURSELF

'Hello, nice to meet you. My name is Dr Smith.'

SET THE SCENE

'I'm sorry to hear that the antidepressants you have tried have not helped very much with the depression.'

'The team thinks that a treatment called ECT, or electroconvulsive therapy, may be helpful in your case.'

FIND OUT WHAT THEY ALREADY KNOW

'Have you heard of ECT before?' 'What do you know about this treatment?'

Be prepared for negative comments that he has heard through the media, Internet or acquaintances:

'Yes, it is true that it doesn't work for everyone, but it can help in depression that hasn't responded to medication.'

INFORMATION ON ECT

Describe the potential benefits and risks.

Explanation

'ECT involves the use of electricity, which induces a fit or seizure while the patient is asleep.'

'The patient is given a very short (minutes) anaesthetic and muscle relaxant.'

'The anaesthetic means that they won't remember the actual procedure.'

'The patient is aware only of going to sleep.'

'At all times, the anaesthetist, psychiatrist and ECT nurses will be present.'

'ECT pads that give the treatment are placed momentarily on the head.'

A usual course of treatment is between 6 and 12 sessions and given twice a week. ECT is usually given to inpatients but sometimes it is given to outpatients. Likelihood of treatment response: two-thirds with antidepressants alone to four-fifths with ECT. ECT is one of the most effective treatments for depression. It is very safe and there is no evidence to date that ECT harms the brain in any way.

The risks are mainly those of having an anaesthetic. Common side effects include headaches, confusion and drowsiness. The greatest concern for many is the association with memory loss.

Memory effects

'Sometimes, people do complain of short-term memory loss, but this is usually temporary and commonly involves only recent things, for example what you had done just before the treatment. Only rarely do people complain of permanent memory problems.'

The vast majority of people return to their baseline cognitive abilities once the course of treatment has finished.

Bilateral ECT seems to work more effectively and more rapidly than unilateral ECT, but it may also induce greater cognitive side effects. If memory is a concern, then it is possible to start treatment with unilateral ECT and then switch to bilateral ECT if there is no significant improvement.

IF THE PATIENT REFUSES OR IS UNDECIDED

Suggest he could think about it and perhaps talk to friends, family or some patients who have had ECT before. He could also visit the ECT suite to speak to the people there.

The patient can refuse ECT treatment at any point (unless being treated under the Mental Health Act). Preparation for ECT requires informed consent from the patient.

ASK WHETHER HE HAS ANY OTHER QUESTIONS

THANK HIM

FOR EXTRA MARKS

Other similar OSCEs reported:
- Discuss the benefits and risks of ECT with this patient who has resistant depression.
- Explain to this relative what happens to patients during ECT.

Unilateral ECT: electrode is placed on the non-dominant side, 4 cm above the mid-point between the external angle of the eye and the auditory meatus. The other electrode is placed 10 cm above the first electrode, above and in line with the meatus on the same side.

Bilateral ECT: on each side, electrodes are placed 4 cm above the mid-point of the line between the external auditory meatus and the lateral angle of the eye.

Neurochemical changes following ECT:
- increased noradrenalin, dopamine and serotonin
- reduced acetylcholine.

ECT also useful in:
- mania
- lethal catatonia
- Parkinson's disease
- NMS.

A therapeutic seizure length is thought to be around 25 seconds on the EEG tracing, or more than 15 seconds of observed physical seizure.

Investigations before ECT/anaesthetic: include FBC, U&E, ECG, and sickle cell screen in African-Caribbean and Mediterranean people.

Mortality for ECT: two per 100 000 treatments.

FURTHER READING

Potter WZ, Rudorfer MV. Electroconvulsive therapy: a modern medical procedure. *N Engl J Med* 1993; 328: 882–3.

STATION 7: PSYCHOSIS

THE EXAMINER'S MARK SHEET	
Communication/rapport	Risk issues
Perceptions	Answering other questions
Thought disorder	Global rating

INTRODUCE YOURSELF

'Hello, nice to meet you. My name is Dr Smith.'

SET THE SCENE

Use open questions to start:
'I wanted to ask whether anything has been troubling you?'
'I was told that you have been having some trouble with your neighbours. Can you tell me what's been happening?'

ASK FOR PERMISSION

'Would that be OK?'

TAKE A HISTORY OF FORMAL THOUGHT DISORDER AND ABNORMAL PERCEPTIONS: KEY AREAS

Formal thought disorder (FTD) is an abnormality in the mechanism of thinking, expressed as abnormal speech. It will soon become apparent during the conversation and is an observational finding.
Any actor would find this difficult to mimic, but be prepared none the less.
You should be able to recognise:

Derailment (loosening of associations, flight of ideas)
Incoherence (word salad, 'knight's move thinking')
Neologisms
Tangentiality

Perceptions

'I would like to ask you some routine questions that we ask of everybody that we see [*normalising*]. Would that be OK?'
'Does your mind ever seem to play tricks on you?'
'Have you been having experiences that you have found difficult to explain?'

'Do you ever *hear* voices or noises when there is no one else about, with nothing else to explain it?'
'What do the voices say?'

'Do you hear one voice or more?'
'Do they talk to each other?'
'Do they talk specifically about you?'
'Are the voices/noises in your mind or can you hear them through your ears [pseudo-hallucinations]'?

Do you ever *see* things, like visions that other people could not see?'
'Do you ever *smell* things [?gas] that other people don't notice?'
'Do you ever *taste* things and find they are strange and unlike other people's experiences?'
'Do you ever *feel* things, like someone touching you, when there is no one there?'

It is important to consider risk here. Ask if she thinks about harming herself or her neighbours.

ASK WHETHER SHE HAS ANY QUESTIONS

THANK HER

FOR EXTRA MARKS

Examples of additional possible questions

Auditory: Do the voices comment on what you do, say or think?
Do they talk to each other about you?
Can you have a conversation with the voices?
Are the voices clear or muffled?
Are the voices of people you recognise?
Are the voices there all the time?
Do these experiences upset you?
Do you believe that what's happening is real or just your mind playing tricks on you?
Visual: Do the things you see occur in your mind or through your eyes?
Did you realise you were 'seeing things'?
How do you explain this?
Were you fully awake or feeling drowsy or tired?

FURTHER READING

Sims A. *Symptoms in the Mind: An Introduction to Descriptive Psychopathology.* London: Balliere Tindall, 2002.

STATION 8: SEROTONIN SYNDROME

THE EXAMINER'S MARK SHEET

Communication	Management
Preferred diagnosis	Answering other questions
Clinical features	Global rating

INTRODUCE YOURSELF

'Hello. My name's John Smith. I'm the senior house officer.' (Here, the actor pretends to be a colleague so slip back into medical mode.)

SET THE SCENE

'I understand this gentleman has become progressively worse over the period of a day since his paroxetine was increased. Do you know what his blood pressure and pulse are? His doctor has excluded physical causes, but do we know what his blood sugar is? Does he appear confused?'

'I'm concerned that this may be serotonin syndrome.'

FIND OUT WHAT THEY ALREADY KNOW

'Have you seen a patient with serotonin syndrome before?'

'Have you heard of this syndrome?'

INFORMATION ON SEROTONIN SYNDROME

Preferred diagnosis is the serotonin syndrome, but infection, metabolic disturbances, substance misuse or withdrawal, and neuroleptic malignant syndrome need to be excluded.

Although usually mild, serotonin syndrome can be quite severe and lead to multi-organ failure and death. It is due to serotonin hyperstimulation.

Ask exactly when the medication was last taken, what the dose was and how many pills were taken.

Exclude an SSRI overdose.

Are other serotonergic medications being taken or prescribed?

Recognised features

According to Sternbach's diagnostic criteria for serotonin syndrome, at least three of the following are needed:

Agitation/restlessness
Sweating
Diarrhoea

Fever
Hyperreflexia
Reduced co-ordination
Mental state change, e.g. confusion, hypomania
Myoclonus
Tremor/shivering

Onset is usually within a few hours of a drug dose and it usually resolves within 24 hours.

PLAN

Explain to the nurse that you would like to see the patient yourself urgently as this could represent an emergency.

Ask whether any results of baseline investigations are available (e.g. urinalysis, FBC, U&E, CRP, ESR, CPK) and explain that you would want to take blood if these tests have not already been done.

Stop any serotonergic medication.

Supportive measures: cooling blankets if pyrexial
                        IV fluids (rehydration)
                        anticonvulsants if fitting
                        antihypertensive if needed
                        reassurance.

Discuss management with a senior colleague (pharmacy drug information) and the medical team, as the patient may need transfer to a medical ward.

Possible helpful medication: benzodiazepines, e.g. clonazepam for myoclonus
                                chlorpromazine for sedative effect
                                cyproheptadine (possible antiserotonergic activity).

ASK WHETHER SHE HAS ANY OTHER QUESTIONS

THANK HER

FOR EXTRA MARKS

Serotonin syndrome is reported with SSRIs, MAOIs, TCAs and other antidepressants.

Often occurs following combination treatment but can happen following monotherapy.

Other reported symptoms include tachycardia, seizures, nausea, vomiting and hypertension.

Other drugs that might be of use include mirtazapine (serotonin 5HT2 and 5HT3 blockade) and propranolol (serotonin 5HT1 and 5HT2 blockade).

For mild cases, drug discontinuation and benzodiazepine cover are often enough.

For more severe cases, major supportive measures are needed.

FURTHER READING

Birmes P, Coppin D, Schmitt L, Lauque D. Serotonin syndrome: a brief review. *Can Med Assoc J* 2003; **168**: 1439–42.

STATION 9: RISK OF ALZHEIMER'S DISEASE

THE EXAMINER'S MARK SHEET	
Communication	Dementia risk
Empathy	Answering other questions
Dementia explanation	Global rating

INTRODUCE YOURSELF

'Hello, nice to meet you. My name is Dr Smith.'

SET THE SCENE

'I've been told you've recently discovered that your mother's memory problems are due to Alzheimer's disease. Is that correct?'

It is important to let the daughter know that you understand that it must be a shock for her and the family, and that it is perfectly natural for her to worry about her mother and the rest of the family.

FIND OUT WHAT SHE ALREADY KNOWS

'Can I ask you what you already know about dementia and Alzheimer's disease?'

INFORMATION ON DEMENTIA

'Dementia is the most serious cause of memory problems. It mainly affects older people. There are several causes, but the commonest is Alzheimer's disease. In this disease, brain cells are replaced by abnormal deposits, leading to a worsening of normal brain functioning.'

This can lead not only to forgetfulness but also to:

Word-finding difficulties
Difficulty with skills such as dressing and using cutlery
Failure of intelligence, judgement and logic
Personality change, e.g. agitation, withdrawal, inappropriateness, apathy
Suspiciousness
Anxiety and depression
Wandering behaviour
Becoming dependent on others for care

Prognosis

'Unfortunately, dementia nearly always gets steadily worse. The forgetfulness of dementia eventually becomes more problematic, so much so that people with dementia can even get lost in familiar surroundings. As the disease progresses, people with dementia start to forget loved ones. The illness usually runs a course of between 5 and 10 years, but this does vary.'

Risk of Alzheimer's disease

'We are all at risk of developing Alzheimer's disease if we live long enough. At the age of 65 years, the risk of developing Alzheimer's disease is approximately 5 per cent. Over the age of 80 years, about one in five people suffer from dementia. However, four out of five people over the age of 80 are not suffering from dementia.'

'The risk can only be approximated. On balance, the risk to first-degree relatives of patients with Alzheimer's disease who developed the disorder at any time up to the age of 85 years is slightly increased. The additional risk to the children of an affected individual is in the region of one in five.'

Genetic testing

Those families with three or more members having early-onset (60 years or younger) Alzheimer's disease should be referred to a specialist clinical geneticist. The great majority of cases, however, are not linked to single gene mutations but are likely due to a number of genetic risk factors and environmental factors. If she is very concerned, then you could offer to refer her.

Ginkgo biloba

Although results are inconsistent, some studies have shown improvement in cognition and function associated with ginkgo biloba. There is little evidence that there is any benefit to those without cognitive impairment. Ginkgo biloba can be bought over the counter, but they should check with their GP if they are on any regular medication (*Cochrane Database Syst Rev* 2002; (4): CD003120).

ASK WHETHER SHE HAS ANY OTHER QUESTIONS

THANK HER

FOR EXTRA MARKS

Let the family know about self-help groups such as the Alzheimer's Society (www.alzheimers.org.uk), Help the Aged (www.helptheaged.org.uk) and Age Concern (www.ageconcern.org.uk).
Offer leaflets made available by the Royal College of Psychiatrists.
Refer early-onset familial dementia to a regional genetics department.
There is no genetic test available for late-onset Alzheimer's disease.

FURTHER READING

Liddell MB, Lovestone S, Owen MJ. Genetic risk of Alzheimer's disease: advising relatives. *Br J Psychiatry* 2001; **178**: 7–11.

STATION 10: BIPOLAR AFFECTIVE DISORDER: ADVICE TO A RELATIVE

THE EXAMINER'S MARK SHEET	
Communication/rapport	BPAD explanation
Empathy	Answering other questions
BPAD features	Global rating

INTRODUCE YOURSELF

'Hello, nice to meet you. My name is Dr Smith.'

SET THE SCENE

'I understand that your son has been in hospital for some time now and has a diagnosis of bipolar affective disorder. You wanted to know about this condition and some advice – is that correct?'

FIND OUT WHAT THEY ALREADY KNOW

'Do you already know anything about BPAD?'

INFORMATION ON BPAD

The relative might ask:

Q: 'What is bipolar affective disorder?'
A: 'We all experience minor changes in our mood from one day to the next or from one week to the next. Generally, our mood is an appropriate response to the events in our lives at the time. However, people who have BPAD tend to have major changes in mood for no obvious reason. They may be extremely excited or happy when there is no reason to be. Vast increases in energy lead to mania or a manic state. At the other extreme is depression, characterised by low mood, reduced levels of energy and loss of interest. In BPAD, the mood can switch between these two mood states. It can be very disruptive to the affected person's life.'

Q: 'What happens between episodes?'
A: 'Both the episodes and the length of time for which people remain well between episodes vary from one person to the next. Some people might have two to three episodes during a lifetime, while others will have four or more episodes a year. Fortunately, with regular medication, we can reduce or even prevent further episodes of the illness.'

Q: 'How common is the disorder?'

A: 'BPAD is quite common. About one in 100 people will develop this illness at some time in their lives, usually starting before the age of 30, although the illness can start after this age.'

Q: 'I've heard that my son can become deluded. Is this true?'

A: 'At more severe points of the illness, your son may or may not suffer from abnormal thinking. Strange and false beliefs, often held with absolute conviction, can occur in a number of conditions, including BPAD. Fortunately, these symptoms do not persist. They are usually treated with antipsychotic medication.'

ASK WHETHER HE HAS ANY OTHER QUESTIONS

THANK HIM

FOR EXTRA MARKS

Recent onset of severe mental illness leads to distress in both the affected individual and the relatives. The actors are often instructed to play such a relative in an upset and agitated manner. It is most important not to forget to be as empathetic as possible. Asking this man whether he understands each point and summarising are considerate things to do and are likely to score more marks.

Offer leaflets made available by the Royal College of Psychiatrists. Let relatives know about support groups such as The Manic Depression Fellowship.

FURTHER READING

Bauer M, Unutzer J, Pincus HA, Lawson WB. Bipolar disorder. NIMH Affective Disorders Workgroup. *Ment Health Serv Res* 2002; 4: 225–9.

STATION 11: BREAKING BAD NEWS/IMPARTING A DIAGNOSIS

THE EXAMINER'S MARK SHEET	
Communication/rapport	Schizophrenia description
Empathy	Answering other questions
Breaking bad news	Global rating

INTRODUCE YOURSELF

'Hello, nice to meet you. My name is Dr Smith.'

SET THE SCENE

Start with 'How are you feeling at the moment?' This is an open way to begin and also invites a dialogue between yourself and the patient.

FIND OUT WHAT THEY ALREADY KNOW

'What have you been told already about why you are in hospital?'
'I want to talk to you about your diagnosis. Would that be OK with you?'

INFORMATION ON BREAKING BAD NEWS

This is an important station, versions of which are nearly always included in the exam – and rightly so, because insensitive news disclosure can have a long-term adverse impact.

Ask the patient who else should be present, e.g. partner, parents.
Ask the patient whether anyone has discussed their probable diagnosis with them.
Find out what the patient wants to know (studies show that different patients have widely differing views on what they would want in this situation).
The patient may or may not want a full description of all the symptoms of the condition (in this case, schizophrenia).
Ask the patient what level of detail you should cover.
Don't beat around the bush: divulge the diagnosis clearly and give time for reaction.

'Having examined your mental state when you first arrived, and also over the course of your admission, we feel you have a diagnosis of schizophrenia.'
'For some people, this will come as a shock. I've come to talk to you about this diagnosis and also to answer your questions and concerns.'

Empathy

Obviously!

Long lectures are overwhelming and confusing. Decide on what you are going to impart to the patient and stick to it.

Ask the patient whether they understand what you are saying and whether they have any questions.

Respond to the patient's feelings

Make sure you do not miss this opportunity. Responding to the patient crying or becoming angry may be part of this OSCE, so be prepared.

If the patient becomes angry with you or starts crying, let the patient vent their anger/sadness. Look as concerned as possible. Comment on their emotional state, e.g. 'I can see how upset you are.'

Start bringing things to a close by talking about follow-up plans, treatment, etc. Ending on a positive but realistic note, e.g. in terms of prognosis, can be helpful. Beware of difficult questions such as 'Am I going to die?' and 'Am I mad?' Use a calm and rational approach, avoiding controversial responses.

ASK WHETHER THEY HAVE ANY OTHER QUESTIONS

THANK THE PATIENT

FOR EXTRA MARKS

As in many stations, the good marks are going to go to those who can display a calm, collected, empathetic nature with the actor. This is a core skill for any psychiatrist. Do this well and the examiner will find it hard to fail you.

This OSCE is an illustration of a general approach to breaking bad news. In reality, the patient/relative is likely to ask about the symptoms, aetiology and prognosis of the illness.

FURTHER READING

Sullivan HS. *The Psychiatric Interview*. New York: Norton, 1954.

Ptacek JT, Eberhardt TL. Breaking bad news: a review of the literature. *J Am Med Assoc* 1996; **276**: 496–502.

STATION 12: HAZARDS OF ALCOHOL MISUSE

THE EXAMINER'S MARK SHEET	
Communication	Social complications
Biological complications	Answering other questions
Psychological complications	Global rating

INTRODUCE YOURSELF

'Hello, nice to meet you. My name is Dr Smith.'

SET THE SCENE

'How are you finding things on the detoxification unit?'
'Can I ask you what you hope to get out of the admission here?'

FIND OUT WHAT HE ALREADY KNOWS

'Are you aware of any problems related to drinking alcohol?'
Poor insight into condition: is this genuine – i.e. he may really believe there is no harm in drinking – or is he in denial (defence mechanism)?
Be empathetic and try to gauge any hostility, as frankly he may not want a lecture.

INFORMATION ON THE HAZARDS OF ALCOHOL

Approach this task by thinking in terms of biological, psychological and social factors.
It can be easier to start with the social and psychological impacts of alcohol misuse in this OSCE. Ask the patient to examine how, for example, alcohol might have impacted upon his relationships and employment. When moving on to biological factors, ask whether he has noticed problems with his liver, stomach, co-ordination, etc. When he acknowledges certain difficulties, enquire what he ascribes this to. Does he consider alcohol to be involved?

Biological
Wernicke's encephalopathy
Mnemonic *CANON*: Confusion/clouding of consciousness
Ataxia
Nystagmus
Ophthalmoplegia
Neuropathy (peripheral neuropathy may be present)

Haemorrhage in brainstem and hypothalamus caused by severe thiamine deficiency (chronic alcohol dependence).

Korsakoff's psychosis
Occurs late.
Key features are short-term memory impairment with confabulation and peripheral neuropathy.
Total recovery rare.

Liver disease
Fat deposition.
Cirrhosis: can drink moderately for years then increase intake and develop cirrhosis after 1–2 years, women recently showing increased incidences. Genetic factors are involved.
Treatments not very successful.
Transplant an option.

Gastrointestinal
Gastritis
Peptic ulcer (ten per cent)
Pancreatitis

Cardiovascular disease
6 units/day associated with rising blood pressure and increased risk of CVA
Cardiac arrhythmias

Sexual impairment

Congenital abnormalities
Fetal alcohol syndrome.

Psychological/psychiatric
Delirium tremens ('DTs'):   tremor
                                   clouding of consciousness
                                   fever, sweating, tachycardia
                                   mortality ten per cent
Alcoholic hallucinosis: hallucinations in clear consciousness
Pathological jealousy
Depression
Neurotic/anxiety disorders

Social harm
Employment problems
Crime
Drunkenness offences/accidents
Economic factors
Disruption of family relationships

ASK WHETHER HE HAS ANY QUESTIONS

THANK HIM

FOR EXTRA MARKS

Good timing during this station is essential. The time should be divided equally into discussing the physical, psychological and social hazards.

FURTHER READING

Gossop M, Marsden J, Stewart D, Kidd T. The National Treatment Outcome Research Study (NTORS): 4–5 year follow-up results. *Addiction* 2003; **98**: 291–303.

EXAM 4

STATION 1

This 54-year-old gentleman has been taking sertraline for 18 months for a moderate depressive episode (F32.01). He ran out of medication 3 days ago as he was unwell and could not get to the general practitioner for a repeat prescription. Since then, he has been feeling 'rotten'. He thinks his cold/flu symptoms have got worse and he has been unable to sleep. He has been dizzy and nauseous and also describes having been tearful.

Explain to the patient the most likely cause of his presentation.
Explain the commonest symptoms of this condition.
Discuss how you plan to help him.

[advice on page 104]

STATION 2

This 59-year-old man has been behaving differently recently, and his wife has expressed concerns to the family doctor. He has a strong family history of late-onset dementia and his GP feels he may have mild cognitive impairment. You see him in an outpatients' clinic.

Assess his frontal lobe function.

[advice on page 106]

STATION 3

Mr Nicholls, a 53-year-old bus-driver, attends the outpatients' department with his wife. She says he has been drinking alcohol heavily since he was dismissed from work a year or so ago.

Assess this gentleman for the features of alcohol-dependence syndrome.

[advice on page 108]

STATION 4

Mr Johnson, diagnosed recently with bipolar affective disorder, is about to be discharged from an acute psychiatric ward.

Advise him on how to cope with any possible relapse in his condition.
Focus on what Mr Johnson needs to do in the event of a relapse.

[advice on page 110]

STATION 5

Mrs Sutherland, a 46-year-old housewife, reports that she has become increasingly anxious at the prospect of leaving her home. Until recently, she was just about able to leave the house and go shopping, although she did so with dread. On a few occasions, she experienced panic attacks when in the shopping centre, and an ambulance was called. She does not feel anxious at home and has now become almost housebound.

Explain to Mrs Sutherland her most likely diagnosis and exclude important differential diagnoses.
Explain how you will help her.

[advice on page 112]

STATION 6

You are in your outpatients' clinic. A 34-year-old woman has been referred to your team by her GP. The patient has been concerned about her weight for many years and believes she is overweight. As a teenager, she was seen by a child psychiatrist, who diagnosed anorexia nervosa. She was never admitted to hospital, but she was extremely underweight and needed specialist treatment. She made a slow but steady recovery and by her twenties needed no further psychiatric intervention. She is a high achiever and works in a high-pressure job, which she feels has led to an abnormal eating pattern once again.

She wants to know whether she has bulimia and, if so, what causes it.

[advice on page 114]

STATION 7

You are seeing this 65-year-old in the outpatients' department. She has a history of anxiety and depression and has been worrying about the results of her brain scan. Your consultant had requested this investigation as the patient had complained recently of poor memory and headache. On clinical examination, there is no obvious abnormal neurology.

Report back to the patient the findings from her scan.
She wants to know what type of brain scan she had and whether there were any risks to her health from such a scan.

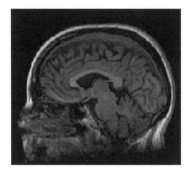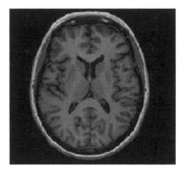

[advice on page 117]

STATION 8

This 45-year-old man has a history of disabling panic attacks. He has told a nurse that he is extremely short of breath and is worried he is dying.

Examine this patient's respiratory system.

[advice on page 120]

STATION 9

The partner of a 46-year-old school teacher has asked to see you. He explains that his girlfriend has been convinced for the past 5 years that she has serious cardiac disease. During this time, she has been investigated by numerous physicians for physical disorders. She reports twice-weekly episodes of sweating, dizziness, tingling sensations in her left arm and a feeling that she is going to die from a heart attack. He says she has become fully preoccupied with the possible outcomes of her 'cardiac disease'.

He asks:

What is the most likely diagnosis?
How did she get it?
What is the most appropriate treatment in this case?

[advice on page 122]

STATION 10

A 29-year-old woman with long-term emotional problems was referred to your clinic by her general practitioner. She is requesting information on CBT and was looking for a referral to a therapist.

Speak to her about CBT.

[advice on page 124]

STATION 11

A 69-year-old woman who lost her husband 7 months ago due to cancer has been attending her GP over the past few weeks. The GP noticed that she is still grieving and is unsure whether this is normal. He would like your opinion.

Assess this woman's response to the loss of her husband.

[advice on page 126]

STATION 12

This is a 53-year old man with a 20-year history of schizophrenia. He is hardly bothered by auditory hallucinations any more and does not have clear delusions as he once did. His next-door neighbour and community psychiatric nurse have become increasingly concerned about him because his personal level of care has declined significantly. He does not interact well with others and he shows few signs of emotion.

Examine him for features of chronic schizophrenia.
The CPN asks how we could help with his negative symptoms.

[advice on page 128]

STATION 1: ANTIDEPRESSANT DISCONTINUATION SYMPTOMS

THE EXAMINER'S MARK SHEET	
Communication/rapport	Simple management
Aetiology and explanation	Answering other questions
Symptoms	Global rating

INTRODUCE YOURSELF

'Hello, my name is Dr Smith. It's nice to meet you.'

SET THE SCENE

'I'm sorry to hear you're not feeling so well. Can you tell me how you've been feeling since you stopped the antidepressant?'

FIND OUT WHAT THEY ALREADY KNOW

'Have you ever before stopped your medication suddenly since you started taking it?'

'Was it ever explained to you that some people can get withdrawal effects if the medication is stopped suddenly?'

INFORMATION ON ANTIDEPRESSANT DISCONTINUATION SYNDROME

Most likely cause

This presentation is likely to represent SSRI discontinuation syndrome. Explain to the patient that his symptoms are probably due to the abrupt cessation of the sertraline medication. Although antidepressants are not addictive, if they are stopped suddenly they can make the patient feel unwell, especially if they have been taking them for 8 weeks or more. Stopping them more gradually over 2–4 weeks usually avoids discontinuation symptoms.

Commonest symptoms

He has a number of recognised features:

Somatic symptoms:	dizziness, nausea, vomiting, fatigue, flu-like symptoms, tremor, insomnia.
Psychological symptoms:	anxiety, agitation, tearfulness, lowered mood, confusion, poor concentration, vivid dreams.

What to do

Give reassurance that the symptoms will pass. Advise him to restart the sertraline, especially if he had been doing well on this drug. If he is prone to forget his medication, then taking an antidepressant with a longer half-life, e.g. fluoxetine, may be appropriate.

Monitor his mental state over the next few weeks to make sure this is not a relapsing depression.

Give advice on taking his medication regularly, as symptoms may occur if medication is stopped suddenly.

ASK WHETHER HE HAS ANY OTHER QUESTIONS

THANK HIM

FOR EXTRA MARKS

Discontinuation symptoms can occur after stopping many different drugs, including SSRIs, MAOIs and TCAs.

The onset is usually within 5 days of stopping treatment.

Discontinuation usually resolves after 2–3 weeks without treatment.

FURTHER READING

Haddad PM. Antidepressant discontinuation syndromes. *Drug Safety* 2001; 24: 183–97.

STATION 2: FRONTAL LOBES

THE EXAMINER'S MARK SHEET	
Communication/rapport	Motor tests
Personality assessment	Primitive reflexes
Verbal tests	Global rating

INTRODUCE YOURSELF
'Hello, nice to meet you. My name is Dr Smith.'

SET THE SCENE
Explain that both his wife and his doctor are concerned about him, and why. Does he think there is a problem?

ASK FOR PERMISSION
Ask him whether it would be OK if you went through some questions and tests that you ask everyone you see.
'Some of the things I'll be asking will be quite difficult, while others will be easier, but try not to worry if you make some mistakes.'
'Let me know if you are uncomfortable at any point or getting too tired.'

CLINICAL PROCEDURE: TEST THE FOLLOWING
Personality
'Have you changed in yourself in any way?'
'In what way?'

Motor sequencing (Luria's test)
Demonstrate the hand sequence – fist, edge, palm – five times and then ask the patient to repeat with both hands (ideally 30 seconds each side).

Verbal fluency
Ask the patient to generate as many words (but not names or places) as possible beginning with the letters F, A and S. Allow 1 minute for each and record all responses.
Depending upon the time available, 1 minute for just one letter would be adequate.

Category fluency
Ask the patient to name, for example, as many animals with four legs in 1 minute as they can.
Record all responses.

Abstract reasoning (proverb interpretation)

Ask the patient to interpret what a proverb might mean, e.g. 'Too many cooks spoil the broth.'

Cognitive estimates

Ask the patient to estimate the following and record the responses:

How many camels are there in Holland?
How tall is the Post Office Tower?

Abstract similarities

Ask the patient in what way the following are similar:

An apple and a banana
A table and a chair

Primitive reflexes

Grasp reflex
Rooting reflex
Palmomental reflex

THANK THE PATIENT

FOR EXTRA MARKS

Features of frontal lobe dysfunction:

Disinhibition, distractibility
Lack of drive
Errors of judgement
Failure to anticipate
Perseveration
Poor adaptation to change
Overfamiliarity
Sexual indiscretion

STATION 3: FEATURES OF ALCOHOL DEPENDENCE

THE EXAMINER'S MARK SHEET	
Communication	Answering other questions
Empathy	Global rating
Features of dependence	

INTRODUCE YOURSELF

'Hello, nice to meet you. My name is Dr Smith.'

SET THE SCENE

'I wanted to speak to you today about alcohol, and in particular your drinking habits.'

ASK FOR PERMISSION

'Would that be OK?'

TAKE A HISTORY OF THE ALCOHOL DEPENDENCE SYNDROME: KEY AREAS

Enquire about the amount, type and units of alcohol consumed.

Stereotyped pattern: non-dependent drinkers drink in accordance with a variety of cues, whereas dependent drinkers drink to avoid symptoms of withdrawal. The drinking repertoire therefore is narrowed.

Salience of drinking behaviour: the dependent drinker will continue to drink despite negative consequences, e.g. financial, familial, physical.

Compulsion to drink: the individual knows that taking a drink is irrational and the action is resisted but, as in the case of compulsions in OCD, further drink is taken.

Increased tolerance to alcohol: physiological and neurochemical changes (more alcohol is needed to achieve the same effect). In later stages, tolerance is lost. This is of unknown aetiology.

Repeated withdrawal symptoms: shaking, trembling, anxiety, physiological craving, vomiting and seizures.

Relief or avoidance of withdrawal symptoms: by repeated drinking. The person may drink throughout the night and on waking in severe cases.

Reinstatement after abstinence: for severe dependence, following a period of abstinence, the previous high levels of alcohol intake and tolerance can be achieved within a number of days.

ASK WHETHER THEY HAVE ANY QUESTIONS

THANK THEM

FOR EXTRA MARKS

Learn to:

Cover all the features of alcohol dependence by asking appropriate questions, and practise them, e.g. (for withdrawal symptoms) 'What would happen if you were to stop drinking?' 'Would you start to feel uncomfortable in any way?'

Calculate the number of units in particular cans and bottles:

$$\frac{\text{Amount of drink in millilitres} \times \text{percentage of alcohol}}{1000}$$

FURTHER READING

Edwards G, Gross M Alcohol dependence: provisional description of a clinical syndrome. *Br Med J* 1976; 1: 1058–61.

STATION 4: BIPOLAR DISORDER: PREVENTING A RELAPSE

THE EXAMINER'S MARK SHEET	
Communication	Advice on relapse prevention
Empathy	Answering other questions
Relapse signature	Global rating

INTRODUCE YOURSELF

'Hello, nice to meet you. My name is Dr Smith.'

SET THE SCENE

'I'm pleased to hear that you are well enough to be discharged. Of course, now it's important that you remain well.'

FIND OUT WHAT HE KNOWS ALREADY

'Has anyone spoken to you about what to do if you feel you are becoming unwell in the future?'

INFORMATION ON RELAPSE PREVENTION

This is a somewhat tricky station without knowing some of the theory behind relapse. The prodromal phase of BPAD is a crucial time, during which small interventions can have a huge impact on the evolution of a full-blown illness. Tell the patient: 'BPAD cannot be prevented, but mood swings can be controlled with medication if it is taken regularly.'

'As with all mental illnesses and other serious conditions, BPAD can affect all aspects of a person's life. Without careful management, it can damage one's self-esteem, relationships and ability to work. This is why it is vital for the individual to try to keep their lives as routine as possible and to let others know when they feel that they are becoming unwell.'

Relapse signature

This is the name given to the pattern of symptoms that arise in an early relapse. In manic relapse, this might include becoming excessively cheerful, overspending or becoming promiscuous. If the patient or people around him can recognise the onset of symptoms, then early intervention might prevent a relapse.

Relapse prevention

'Take medication regularly.'
'Eat a balanced diet and at regular times.'
'Exercise at regular times.'

Consistent sleep: 'Spend nights in your bedroom, even if you are not sleeping. A simple repetitive card game like patience may help with sleep.'
'Avoid the use of alcohol and illicit drugs' (stimulants).
Reduce stress at home and in the workplace: 'Ask family and friends to remain calm if you are becoming unwell. It will help if they try to ignore silly remarks or pranks.'
'Avoid arguments and confrontations.'
Reduce stimulation if a manic phase is developing: 'Avoid crowds, parties and listening to loud fast music.'
It is good advice not to leave money and credit-cards lying around (family members and house sharers).
'Learn to relax.'
'Progressive muscle relaxation is a useful technique.'
'Use a structured problem-solving technique.'
'Have a structured routine to the day.'
'Seek treatment as soon as you or others notice a depressive/manic episode evolving.'

PROFESSIONAL INPUT

It is important to have a care plan drawn up to which he can refer. This will include advice on what to do should his mood be destabilising:

Contact the community psychiatric nurse, psychiatrist or GP for assessment (possible drug changes, dosage alteration, blood levels).
Re-admission/community management.

ASK WHETHER HE HAS ANY OTHER QUESTIONS

THANK HIM

FOR EXTRA MARKS

Increase 'useful' activities.
It is important that family members do not try to stop all activities.
Careful prior planning of relaxing and constructive activities will be helpful.

FURTHER READING

Vieta E, Colom F. Psychological interventions in bipolar disorder: from wishful thinking to an evidence-based approach. *Acta Psychiatr Scand Suppl* 2004; (422): 34–8.

STATION 5: AGORAPHOBIA

THE EXAMINER'S MARK SHEET	
Communication	Basic treatment options
Diagnosis	Answering other questions
Agoraphobia explanation	Global rating

INTRODUCE YOURSELF

'Hello, nice to meet you. My name is Dr Smith.'

SET THE SCENE

'I've heard a little bit about what's been happening to you. Am I right in saying that the thought of leaving your home makes you the most anxious?'

'It must be very distressing for you not to be able to leave the house.'

FIND OUT WHAT SHE ALREADY KNOWS

'Has anyone told you what they think is going on in your case or discussed a diagnosis with you?'

'Do you know anything about a condition called agoraphobia?'

INFORMATION ON AGORAPHOBIA

Diagnosis

Agoraphobia is the most likely diagnosis. Explain what this means in understandable terms to the patient:

'Agoraphobia is an anxiety disorder associated with an uneasiness, fear or dread about leaving familiar places. The affected individual might be frightened to travel, particularly on public transport, or to be in crowded places. There is an association between the physical symptoms of anxiety and panic attacks. It is a condition related to anxiety, depression, panic and other phobias.'

'Initially, a person may have a panic attack for no particular reason. Then a real fear develops that it may happen again, and the person avoids those situations that remind them of the previous panic attacks. Because the panic attacks are scary and embarrassing, the person tries to avoid what they think caused the panic attack.'

Differential diagnosis

Other causes of anxiety must be considered (social phobia, specific phobia, panic disorder, generalised anxiety disorder).

Social phobia, for example, can lead the individual to avoid leaving the house for fear of being scrutinised by others. In agoraphobia, individuals fear having a panic attack.

Psychosis
An individual may avoid public places because of delusional beliefs, e.g. that they may be harmed.

Depression
An affected individual might feel too low in mood, energy-deplete and unmotivated to leave their home. This may or may not be associated with anxiety. (Enquire about their mood.)

Obsessive–compulsive disorder
This can lead to fear of contamination in public places and, hence, avoidance of the area.

Managing agoraphobia

Educate about the nature of anxiety and the nature of the fight or flight response.

Educate also about the role of hyperventilation in anxiety. Breathing control and slow breathing exercises are very important.

Graded exposure to the feared situation will be the mainstay of treatment, which you or a psychologist will perform.

SSRIs can be prescribed.

ASK WHETHER SHE HAS ANY OTHER QUESTIONS

THANK HER

FOR EXTRA MARKS

Agoraphobia with or without panic disorder affects two per cent of the population in any one year.

Peaks in mid to late twenties.

Twenty per cent of patients have an associated anxiety disorder.

The Fear Questionnaire was developed to monitor change in phobic individuals (*Behav Res Ther* 1979; 17: 263–7).

SUPPORT GROUPS

No Panic: www.nopanic.org.uk
Open Door Association (Agoraphobia): 447 Pensby Road, Heswall, Wirral, Merseyside L61 9PQ
National Phobics Society: www.phobics-society.org.uk

FURTHER READING

Shear MK, Cassano GB, Frank E, *et al.* The panic-agoraphobic spectrum: development, description, and clinical significance. *Psychiatr Clin North Am* 2002; 25: 739–56.

STATION 6: BULIMIA NERVOSA

THE EXAMINER'S MARK SHEET	
Communication	Aetiology
Current eating habits	Answering other questions
Bulimia explanation	Global rating

INTRODUCE YOURSELF

'Hello, nice to meet you. My name is Dr Smith.'

SET THE SCENE

'Your doctor has told me that you are concerned about your pattern of eating at the moment. Is that right?'

'Could you tell me about your current eating pattern?'

FIND OUT WHAT THEY ALREADY KNOW

'Your GP tells me that you think you might have bulimia. Do you know much about bulimia nervosa (BN)?'

INFORMATION ON BULIMIA NERVOSA

Making the diagnosis

Remember to speak in lay terms. You should take a food and weight history and try to cover the following points (ICD-10 criteria for BN):

Persistent preoccupation with eating and a craving for food

Overeating large amounts of food in short periods of time (bingeing)

An attempt to counteract fattening effects of food by one or more of vomiting, purging, starvation and drugs (appetite suppressants, thyroid analogues, diuretics, insulin)

Psychopathology: morbid dread of fatness

Low self-induced weight threshold

Often a history of AN

Other features of BN may include normal weight and irregular periods.

Aetiology

'There are a number of contributing factors that are thought to be risk factors for the development of eating disorders, including bulimia nervosa.'

Social

Cultural emphasis on slimness
Media pressure
Particular association with certain professions
Fashion for dieting
Sense of control over your life when dieting/restricting calories

Family

Eating disorders can run in the family. First-degree relatives of individuals with BN have an increased risk of an eating disorder.

An environment in which members of the family have had issues with food or been critical of eating, weight or body shape often contributes to eating disorders.

Depression

Often, people will turn to food when thy feel low. It is possible that BN starts off in this way, because of a feeling of unhappiness. The guilt associated with bingeing is then associated with vomiting or purging.

Life events

'Sometimes, upsetting events, like the end of a relationship, can trigger bulimia.'

Serious life events can trigger bulimia onset in up to 70 per cent of bulimia cases (*Psychol Med* 1997; **27**: 523–30).

History of childhood (sexual) abuse and parental neglect, loss, indifference and separation have all been suggested as risk factors.

Personality

'Some of us have parts of our personalities that might make us more likely to develop bulimia nervosa.'

Presence of certain traits, including perfectionism, impulsivity, mood lability, thrill-seeking and dysphoria associated with rejection.

ASK WHETHER SHE HAS ANY OTHER QUESTIONS

THANK HER

FOR EXTRA MARKS

Borderline personality traits are more common in BN than in AN.

$$BMI = \frac{\text{(weight in kilograms)}}{\text{(height in metres)}^2}.$$

Differential diagnosis of weight loss: physical (hyperthyroid, malignancy, malabsorption), AN, BN, depression, OCD, personality.

Fifty per cent of people with AN also meet the criteria for BN.

FURTHER READING

Cooper P, Fairburn C. *Bulimia Nervosa and Binge Eating: A Guide to Recovery*. London: Constable & Robinson, 1993.

Fairburn C. *Overcoming Binge Eating*. New York: Guildford Press, 1995.

STATION 7: MRI INTERPRETATION

THE EXAMINER'S MARK SHEET	
Communication/rapport	MRI risks
Empathy	Answering other questions
MRI interpretation	Global rating

INTRODUCE YOURSELF

'Hello, nice to meet you. My name is Dr Smith.'

SET THE SCENE

'Am I right in thinking you have been having some worries since your brain scan? This is entirely understandable.'
'What has been worrying you?'

FIND OUT WHAT SHE ALREADY KNOWS

'Do you already know anything about MRI scans or magnetic resonance imaging?'

INFORMATION ON MRI

Interpreting the MRI (similar for CT)

Use lay terms to explain the scan findings to a patient. A variant of this OSCE would involve discussing the findings with a colleague.
Check the scan is:

Named
Dated
Orientated correctly

Comment on whether the image is axial (as if looking from above/below), sagittal (sideways on) or coronal (from the front).
Note any obvious abnormalities (e.g. cortical atrophy or an intracerebral mass such as a tumour/abscess). Others might include cerebral shift, calcification (better on CT), high-signal change, plaques (demyelination) and haemorrhage.
Look systematically at the main structures:

Bone (better in CT)
Lateral ventricles (enlarged or displaced?)
Cerebral cortices and cerebellum (white and grey matter)
Sulci (reduction?) and gyri (increased?)

When speaking to the patient, show them the scan if possible.

'Well, here is the MRI of your brain. The first thing to say is your brain looks normal, which is very good news.'

Ask the patient whether she would like a more detailed explanation. If yes, go through the main structures (as above) and explain in very simple lay terms.

'I am not a radiologist and will, of course, get one of my colleagues to look at this as well.'

The example MRI scan here is normal.

Scan type

'You had an MRI scan. This stands for magnetic resonance imaging.'

She may ask for a little more detail (keep it simple!):

'The MR image is very good at looking at soft tissues like the brain.'

'It allows high-resolution (quality) images of the different types of brain tissue (white and grey matter) and can usually show us quite clearly whether there are any obvious abnormalities.'

'MRI also allows us to look at the brain in three different planes (directions), which means that we get good views of the brain from different angles.'

Risks

MRI has the advantage of avoiding X-ray radiation exposure.

There are no known side effects.

Risk is associated with metal inside the body, such as surgical staples, pacemakers and metallic plates.

It is painless (as she knows).

One of the main disadvantages (as she may have discovered) is that lying inside the scanner can feel quite claustrophobic.

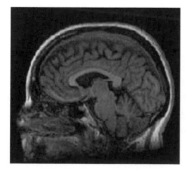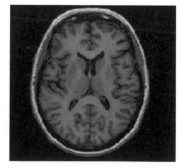

ASK WHETHER SHE HAS ANY OTHER QUESTIONS

THANK HER

FOR EXTRA MARKS

EXAMPLE PRESENTATION TO A COLLEAGUE (not the MRI shown)

'This is an axial brain MR image of Mrs Jones, a 65-year-old woman, taken on the twenty-fourth of June, 2005. The most obvious abnormality is a large circumscribed mass in the right frontal lobe, which could be consistent with a primary or secondary tumour. It appears to be surrounded by a degree of high-intensity signal [white/bright on MRI], which would fit with associated oedema . . .'

Comment on the possible differential diagnosis if abnormal.

MRI uses magnetism, radio waves and a computer to create detailed images of body tissues (the physics is complicated).
MRI scanning is noisy and involves lying in a confined space.
MRI images water and not calcium. Subsequently, seeing bone (white) clearly is likely to mean that you are looking at a CT scan.
MRI produces high signals from fat (bright) and low signals from bone.
A concise and to-the-point description of the image will give the examiners confidence.

THE CT

Useful for looking at bony structures.
Used when MRI cannot be used.
Less claustrophobic, but exposes the patient to ionising radiation.

STATION 8: RESPIRATORY SYSTEM

THE EXAMINER'S MARK SHEET

Communication/rapport	Percussion
Inspection	Auscultation
Palpation	Global rating

INTRODUCE YOURSELF

'Hello, nice to meet you. My name is Dr Smith.'

SET THE SCENE

'I can see you are short of breath so I would like to examine your chest and lungs.'

ASK FOR PERMISSION

'Would that be OK?'
'I would normally ask for a chaperone, but are you alright to continue?'
'Let me know if you are uncomfortable at any point.'

CLINICAL PROCEDURE

The patient should be sitting comfortably (ideally, on an examination couch).
Remember: inspection, palpation, percussion and auscultation.
Expose the patient's chest.

Inspection

Observe the breathing pattern and respiratory rate.
Is the patient emaciated or coughing?

Examine for:

Clubbing (hands)
Peripheral (extremities) or central cyanosis (lips and tongue)
Cervical lymphadenopathy
Eyes (Horner's syndrome causes ptosis and constricted pupil – sympathetic chain involvement in carcinoma of the lung)
Chest-wall deformities, intercostal recession, scars (this will depend on the gender of the patient and the need for a chaperone): be tactful!

Palpation

Trachea: position, deviation?
Chest wall: feel for tactile vocal fremitus (ask patient to say 'ninety-nine').

Chest expansion: ask the patient to take a deep breath and feel expansion on both sides (normally 5 cm).

Percussion
Compare right with left on both sides and all lung fields anteriorly and posteriorly.

Auscultation
Listen for the presence of:

Vesicular breath sounds (normal)
Bronchial breathing
Vocal resonance
Added sounds (wheeze, crackles, rub, stridor)

THANK THE PATIENT

FOR EXTRA MARKS
Explain the procedure to the patient as you go alone, so the examiner knows what you are doing, e.g. 'I'm just checking your hands. Sometimes the nails can change shape if there are lung problems. Have you noticed this?'

CAUSES OF CLUBBING
Pulmonary: bronchial carcinoma
            chronic pulmonary scpsis
            fibrosing alveolitis
Cardiac: congenital cyanotic heart disease
            bacterial endocarditis
Other: familial
            idiopathic
            inflammatory bowel disease

STATION 9: HYPOCHONDRIACAL DISORDER

THE EXAMINER'S MARK SHEET

Communication

Diagnosis

Aetiology

Treatment approaches

Answering other questions

Global rating

INTRODUCE YOURSELF

'Hello, nice to meet you. My name is Dr Smith.'

Only the patient's partner is seeing you.

Make sure the patient has given permission to talk about her case.

SET THE SCENE

'Your partner appears to have been suffering from the belief that she has a heart problem for a long time. Is that correct?'

'That must have been difficult for both of you.'

'Are there any other worries or anxieties that she complains of to you?'

FIND OUT WHAT THEY ALREADY KNOW

'Have you heard of a condition called hypochondriacal disorder?'

'What do you already know about it?'

INFORMATION ON HYPOCHONDRIASIS

Diagnosis

'Hypochondriasis is a preoccupation with the possibility of at least one serious illness, which persists despite medical reassurance to the contrary.'

The diagnosis must be differentiated from certain conditions, so ask him relevant questions about the following:

Somatisation disorder

Depression

Delusional disorder

Anxiety/panic disorder

Refusing the advice and reassurance of a number of doctors is a classic feature and is required for a definitive diagnosis (ICD-10).

The belief is held strongly, but these patients are not delusional.

Aetiology

The origins of this illness can be based on a cognitive-behavioural model, whereby there is a misinterpretation of harmless physical symptoms as evidence of serious illness.

This leads to anxiety, which leads to seeking reassurance, avoidance and bodily checking (an increased preoccupation with the body), which leads to further self-investigation for symptoms, which then leads to further misinterpretation of benign symptoms.

Treatment

Often, the patient refuses psychiatric treatment.
Due to the chronicity of such conditions, treatment can be difficult.

CBT has been shown to be helpful in some cases:
-   Self-monitor for hypochondriacal symptoms and reattribute the thoughts/symptoms.
-   Exposure and response prevention.
-   Identification and alternatives are sought for faulty assumptions.
Group psychotherapy can be useful.
Medication can be tried but is thought to be of limited benefit.

ASK WHETHER HE HAS ANY OTHER QUESTIONS

THANK HIM

FOR EXTRA MARKS

Men : women 1 : 1.
Usually presents in the second or third decade.

If you are asked to see the patient in this station, you will need to ask:

Do you worry about your physical health?
What do you think is wrong with you?
How many doctors have you seen in the past 2 years?
Has medical reassurance convinced you that nothing is wrong?
Do you feel relieved when you are told that everything is OK?

FURTHER READING

Abramowitz JS, Schwartz SA, Whiteside SP. A contemporary conceptual model of hypochondriasis. *Mayo Clin Proc* 2002; **77**: 1323–30.

STATION 10: EXPLAINING COGNITIVE-BEHAVIOURAL THERAPY

THE EXAMINER'S MARK SHEET	
Communication	CBT sessions explained
Brief history of complaint	Answering other questions
CBT explanation	Global rating

INTRODUCE YOURSELF

'Hello, nice to meet you. My name is Dr Smith.'

SET THE SCENE

'Your GP has written to me and tells me you are interested in cognitive-behavioural therapy. Is that right?'
'Have you ever had psychotherapy or CBT before?'
Ask her briefly what she thinks CBT is likely to help her with. You do not want to make an inappropriate referral.

FIND OUT WHAT SHE ALREADY KNOWS

'Can you tell me what you've heard or know about CBT?'

INFORMATION ON CBT

'CBT stands for cognitive-behavioural therapy. It's a talking therapy.'
In the treatment, the therapist works with the patient on unhelpful automatic thoughts and/or behaviours that are causing or contributing to the complaint. CBT combines two very effective kinds of psychotherapy – cognitive therapy and behaviour therapy. These are very effective for a number of psychological conditions.
'*Cognitive therapy* teaches you how certain thinking patterns are causing your symptoms, by distorting your opinion of what's actually going on in your life. This pattern of thinking might be making you feel anxious, depressed or angry for no good reason.'
'For example, if a friend doesn't invite someone to a party, then the person might start by thinking they weren't invited because they're not fun to be with. This leads to the thought that nobody likes them and then on to the thought that they'll always be alone and disliked. The therapist works on such negative assumptions.'
'*Behaviour therapy* helps you weaken the connections between troublesome situations and your usual reactions to them – reactions such as fear, depression, anger and self-defeating behaviour. It also teaches you better control of your thinking and physical responses, so you can feel better and think more clearly.'

CBT sessions

It is a here-and-now therapy.

There are typically 8–20 sessions over a few months.

The therapy is collaborative with the therapist.

Weekly sessions involve problem-solving and reviewing diary-keeping and homework set from the last session.

Research evidence shows that CBT is useful in depression and anxiety.

Patients can continue on medication during the course of the therapy.

ASK WHETHER SHE HAS ANY OTHER QUESTIONS

THANK HER

FOR EXTRA MARKS

Don't overwhelm the patient with technical terms.

Patients who have difficulty forming a working alliance with a therapist are likely to do poorly with CBT.

The cognitive-behavioural therapist takes a directive, active and problem-oriented approach, unlike the psychodynamic therapist, who allows a patient-led approach.

FURTHER READING

Hawton K. *Cognitive Behaviour Therapy for Psychiatric Problems: A Practical Guide.* Oxford: Oxford University Press, 1989.

Beck AT. Cognitive models of depression. *J Cogn Psychother* 1987; 1: 5–37.

STATION 11: GRIEF REACTION

THE EXAMINER'S MARK SHEET

Communication/rapport	Features of abnormal grief
Empathy	Answering other questions
History of grief	Global rating

INTRODUCE YOURSELF

'Hello, nice to meet you. My name is Dr Smith.'

SET THE SCENE

'I was sorry to hear about your husband passing away recently.'
'I wanted to find out how you had been feeling since this happened.'

ASK FOR PERMISSION

'Would that be OK?'

TAKE A HISTORY OF HER GRIEF REACTION: KEY AREAS

Try to elicit the features of grief from your history.
The literature has yet to show consensus on a clear definition of normal and abnormal or complicated grief reactions. However, the symptoms of normal grief are as follows:

Preoccupation with the deceased (this occurs in all cases of grief)
Pining or searching
Somatic responses, e.g. crying, disturbed sleep and appetite
Mummification, i.e. leaving the person's bedroom or belongings intact, exactly as they were before death
Hallucinations or illusions of the deceased – common in normal individuals and considered part of the normal grieving process. Can be in any modality but most commonly auditory
Guilt

Resolution follows. The bereaved person might always be affected by the loss but will resume old or new activities.

Abnormal grief reaction

The normal process is thought to last 6 months. Strictly, anything beyond this should be considered abnormal, but the cut-off is not accepted widely. Delayed grief, where symptoms take longer than normal to develop (> 2 weeks), is also considered abnormal.

Characteristic features

General inability to function
Excessive hallucinatory experiences (more bizarre and varied hallucinations)
Protracted mummification – the whole house may remain exactly as it was, e.g.
the table may be set for the deceased. This behaviour does not lessen with time
Thoughts of self-harm and suicide (again, this can be normal in the initial stages
of grief but if prolonged can be a worrying feature)

Other features can include:

Acquiring features or symptoms of the deceased's final illness
Retaining an idealised view of the deceased

In this case, an antidepressant is warranted if features of depression are evident.

ASK WHETHER SHE HAS ANY QUESTIONS

THANK HER

FOR EXTRA MARKS

Once again, the candidate who can appear naturally empathetic will gain the
most marks.
A grief reaction does not only occur through the loss of a person: it can
occur following the loss of a pet or a limb.
Abnormal grief is more likely following a sudden death or suicide, if the
bereaved person was dependent on the deceased, if there is a history of
previous psychiatric illness, or if there is an inability to grieve because of
dependants, e.g. children.
Differentiating grief from depression can be tricky. The length of the
presentation is important but so too are the differences in clinical features. If
asked in an OSCE to differentiate between the two, use the ICD-10 or DSM-IV
criteria for depression to help you.

PSYCHOLOGICAL TREATMENT

Grief counselling
Grief therapy

FURTHER READING

Bonanno GA, Kaltman S. The varieties of grief experience. *Clin Psychol Rev*
2001; 21: 705–34.

STATION 12: CHRONIC SCHIZOPHRENIA

THE EXAMINER'S MARK SHEET	
Communication	Simple management approach
Empathy	Answering other questions
Negative features	Global rating

INTRODUCE YOURSELF

'Hello, nice to meet you. My name is Dr Smith.'

SET THE SCENE

'I wanted to talk to you about how you have been feeling recently.'

ASK FOR PERMISSION

'Would that be OK?'
'I've been asked to see you because your nurse has been concerned about you.'
'Is anything worrying or upsetting you at the moment?'
This patient is likely to be quiet, withdrawn and possibly difficult to understand.
Be patient with him, speak clearly and offer reassurance where appropriate.

TAKE A HISTORY OF CHRONIC SCHIZOPHRENIA: KEY AREAS

Features of chronic schizophrenia

Try to elicit the following features (ICD-10 criteria for a diagnosis of residual schizophrenia):

Psychomotor slowing
Underactivity
Blunting of affect
Passivity and lack of initiative
Poverty of quantity or content of speech
Reduced facial expression and eye contact
Poor self-care and social performance

There should have been at least one previous clear-cut psychotic episode reaching the diagnostic criteria for schizophrenia.
There should have been a minimum of 1 year where there has been a significant reduction in the intensity of delusions and hallucinations and the negative syndrome is present.

MANAGING NEGATIVE SYMPTOMS

Consider a biological/psychological/social approach:

Biological

Medication: in the first instance, you would consider atypical neuroleptics. Many people claim efficacy of atypical neuroleptics against negative symptoms compared with older drugs. The best evidence exists for amisulpride for primary negative symptoms.

Psychological

Psychotherapeutic assessment for CBT: it is reported that people with chronic schizophrenia are no more cognitively impaired than other schizophrenic diagnostic subgroups, and so they may be suitable. However, motivation may be a problem.

Social

Need increased prompting and support with hygiene and self-care.
Additional help needed with bill payments, food, shopping, etc.
Family/carers to be educated and advised on the disorder and their possible input.
Patients may require admission to hospital or a supported environment if they represent a risk to themselves through self-neglect.

ASK WHETHER HE HAS ANY OTHER QUESTIONS

THANK HIM

FOR EXTRA MARKS

If time allows, exclude dementia, an organic syndrome and chronic depression.

Try to establish whether negative symptoms are primary or secondary:

Primary: transient or enduring.

Secondary to: positive symptoms: as a consequence of paranoid symptoms
                depression: social withdrawal
                EPSE: bradykinesia, etc.

The chronic syndrome is often characterised by thought disorder, underactivity, reduced drive, social withdrawal and emotional apathy.

The earlier a psychotic disorder is treated, the less likely the person is to go on to develop a negative syndrome.

FURTHER READING

Carpenter WT, Jr. The treatment of negative symptoms: pharmacological and methodological issues. *Br J Psychiatry Suppl* 1996; (29): 17–22.

Waddington JL, Youssef HA, Kinsella A. Sequential cross-sectional and 10-year prospective study of severe negative symptoms in relation to duration of initially untreated psychosis in chronic schizophrenia. *Psychol Med* 1995; 25: 849–57.

EXAM 5

STATION 1

This 35-year-old woman took a large paracetamol overdose several days ago. She has developed fulminant hepatic failure and needs an urgent liver transplantation. The physicians have told you that she is alert and not delirious. They have asked you to assess her as they want to make sure she has capacity before transplantation.

Assess this patient's capacity.
Can she consent to treatment?

[advice on page 136]

STATION 2

A fitness instructor of 24 years, James Dawson is currently admitted having had a hypomanic episode. He experienced his first hypomanic episode at 18 years of age. His father was diagnosed with bipolar disorder as a young man and was treated with lithium to good effect.

Mr Dawson is looking for information about lithium and is curious about his suitability for the treatment.

[advice on page 138]

STATION 3

This patient complains of chest pain.

Examine their cardiovascular system.

[advice on page 141]

STATION 4

Ms Martin, a 28-year-old bank clerk, describes experiencing recurrent and unpredictable attacks of anxiety or panic. The attacks start suddenly, are extremely distressing and last for a few minutes, sometimes longer. She says that the episodes can happen anywhere.

Discuss the most likely diagnosis and the differential diagnosis.
How will you manage this woman?

[advice on page 143]

STATION 5

This 73-year-old man had a cerebrovascular accident several years ago, from which he made a good physical recovery. His GP referred him to psychiatric services with a possible depressive episode. The specialist registrar asks you to see the man in the day hospital, as he has commitments elsewhere. From the notes available, you notice that in a cognitive assessment 2 years ago, the man drew only half a clock face.

Assess his parietal lobe function.

[advice on page 145]

STATION 6

This gentleman presented to the A&E department in the early hours of the morning. He remains slightly drowsy, but he has been cleared from a medical perspective. The nursing staff have been too busy to gather any personal information from the man but mention that he smells ethanolic.

Assess this gentleman.

[advice on page 147]

STATION 7

This 30-year-old postman has given himself up to the police, claiming he can 'no longer hide from them'. The police are concerned about his mental state and inform you that he has been mumbling to himself. He appears to be exhausted and distractible.

Assess his mental state.

Do not enquire about his past history.

[advice on page 149]

STATION 8

A 28-year-old woman has been unable to return to work for 6 months following a flu-like illness. The acute illness has resolved but she remains exhausted and achy. She is referred to your clinic, as various doctors have been unable to find a physical cause.

Discuss the most likely diagnosis.
How will you begin to help this woman?

[advice on page 151]

STATION 9

This 75-year-old woman has recently made a will. You have been asked to see her because her children are concerned about her ability to construct an appropriate will. They have raised her 'failing memory and change in behaviour'.

Assess her testamentary capacity.

[advice on page 154]

STATION 10

Give advice to this patient who takes lithium for a bipolar affective disorder and is planning to travel to a tropical country.

[advice on page 156]

STATION 11

Mr Stanley, a patient of yours, is due to receive ECT in a few days. As part of his preparation for treatment, you requested a chest X-ray. The X-ray is shown below.

Your consultant asks you to comment on the film.

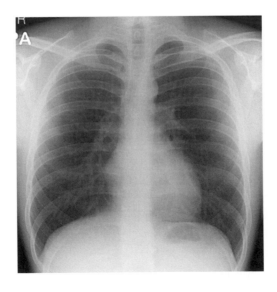

[advice on page 158]

STATION 12

This woman is attending the outpatients' department following instruction from her family doctor. Her doctor informs you that the patient is convinced that Robbie Williams is in love with her. The doctor, who assumed she was joking, made a sarcastic comment and was shocked by the hostile response that it provoked.

Take a history of erotomania.

[advice on page 160]

STATION 1: CAPACITY

THE EXAMINER'S MARK SHEET	
Communication	Consent to treatment
Empathy	Answering other questions
Capacity assessment	Global rating

INTRODUCE YOURSELF

'Hello, my name is Dr Smith. I'm one of the psychiatrists.'

SET THE SCENE

Explain that you are a psychiatrist and that you have been asked by the doctors looking after her to talk to her.

ASK FOR PERMISSION

'Would that be OK?'

This is a very sensitive case where you must show the examiner that you can be empathetic.

Ask whether she remembers the events that led to the overdose and how she feels about it now:

Does she regret the overdose?
Does she wish she had died?
Does she understand that she needs a transplant, and why?
Does she understand what will happen if she does not have a transplant?

ASSESS THIS PATIENT'S CAPACITY: KEY AREAS

Capacity requires the following three criteria to be fulfilled:

Can she understand and retain information on the treatment proposed, its indications, benefits and risks, and the consequences of non-treatment?
She must be shown to believe that information.
She must be able to weigh up the information to arrive at a conclusion.

Consent to treatment

Treating without first obtaining consent in situations in which it would have been appropriate to gain consent can be considered as criminal battery.

A patient's consent for treatment becomes valid when three conditions are fulfilled:

The physician has given the patient adequate information to permit a rational treatment consent or refusal. (You should explain that the physicians are in a better position to do this in this case – the hepatologists or surgeons should discuss the common but non-serious as well as less common but more serious implications of treatment.)

The patient possesses the capacity to make medical decisions (this will already be established from the above).

The treatment consent or refusal is made freely without coercion by other people or agencies.

ASK WHETHER SHE HAS ANY QUESTIONS

THANK HER

FOR EXTRA MARKS

The capacity to consent is called 'competence'.

The more dangerous and invasive a treatment, the greater is the requirement to obtain explicit informed consent.

A signature on a form is not in itself consent. Informed consent is an ongoing process between the doctor and patient, in which the doctor explains and answers the patient's questions.

It is often useful to have the opinion of more than one doctor with regard to capacity, especially in such important cases.

FURTHER READING

Buchanan A. Mental capacity, legal competence and consent to treatment. *J R Soc Med* 2004; **97**: 415–20.

STATION 2: LITHIUM ADVICE

THE EXAMINER'S MARK SHEET	
Communication	Suitability issues
Empathy	Answering other questions
Lithium explanation	Global rating

INTRODUCE YOURSELF

'Hello, nice to meet you. My name is Dr Smith.'

SET THE SCENE

'I've been told you would like some information on lithium treatment. Is that correct?'

'Your father took lithium. Can you remember what that involved?'

FIND OUT WHAT HE ALREADY KNOWS

'Can I ask you what you already know about lithium treatment?'

The patient's response will give you some leads on where to go next.

It is preferable that the interaction with the patient appears natural and comfortable. Try to avoid launching into a textbook recital of everything there is to know about lithium. However, it is important to cover some key points.

INFORMATION ON LITHIUM: SUITABLE OR UNSUITABLE?

Suitable

Illness

'Lithium is used for a number of conditions, including bipolar affective disorder, but also mania, hypomania and recurrent depression. It is a tried and tested medication that has been used successfully for many years.'

In an otherwise uncomplicated case, lithium use can be appropriate treatment for BPAD. Lithium is often considered in BPAD where there have been two illnesses within 2 years or three illnesses in 5 years.

Poor treatment response

Enquire about other mood stabilisers. Has he taken sodium valproate, for example, and found it to be unhelpful? Poor response to other treatments may make lithium a sensible choice.

Can tolerate drug and monitoring

'Lithium is not the easiest of medications to take. The main reasons for this are the side effects and the blood tests. However, if you are OK with the blood tests and accept mild side effects if you get any, then you'll probably get on well with lithium.'

'We require regular blood tests to monitor the lithium serum levels, and kidney and thyroid function. We also need an ECG (trace of the heart) before treatment is started. We monitor the thyroid gland because it can, usually after many years of treatment, become underactive. Lithium can also affect kidney function, but again this is usually after a number of years. More common side effects include mild gastrointestinal symptoms, tremor and mild thirst; others include polyuria and weight gain.'

You will need to explain that the lithium levels in the blood need to be kept within a certain range: too low and there is limited therapeutic value, but too high and there is a risk of toxicity.

'I notice you are a fitness instructor. Causes of dehydration, such as vomiting, diarrhoea or indeed prolonged periods of exercise, can increase the blood lithium levels, which can lead to lithium toxicity. You would need to ensure that you maintained hydration at work. We will give you a leaflet that explains more about lithium and how to avoid running into problems.'

Family history
His father's positive response might predict a similar response.

Unsuitable

Medical health
If he suffers from renal impairment, thyroid disease, cardiac disease or sodium imbalance, e.g. in Addison's disease, then lithium may not be suitable.

Drug interactions
Enquire about regular medications taken. The dangers of toxicity and interactions with other medications, e.g. diuretics and NSAIDs, should be explained. This may mean that lithium treatment is best avoided.

Unable to tolerate side effects
Despite the efficacy of lithium, some people cannot put up with its side effects.

Unable to tolerate monitoring
The monitoring is unacceptable to some people, who may prefer alternative treatments.

ASK WHETHER HE HAS ANY OTHER QUESTIONS

THANK HIM

FOR EXTRA MARKS

Know the basics:

The need for blood tests and the potential side effects are the essentials.
Lithium is usually prescribed in a single dose at night.
Caution about side effects.
Warn about lithium toxicity.

PRE-LITHIUM WORK-UP

Baseline investigation of renal function
ECG
Thyroid function tests

Lithium treatment cards give advice on how to take the drug, monitoring and side effects.
Patients should remain on lithium for more than 5 years only if benefits persist.

FURTHER READING

Cookson J. Lithium: balancing risks and benefits. *Br J Psychiatry* 1997; **178**: 120–24.

STATION 3: CARDIOVASCULAR EXAMINATION

THE EXAMINER'S MARK SHEET	
Communication/rapport	Percussion
Inspection	Auscultation
Palpation	Global rating

INTRODUCE YOURSELF

'Hello, nice to meet you. My name is Dr Smith.'

SET THE SCENE

'Are you still having chest pain? Can you show me where it hurts? I would like to examine your heart.'

ASK FOR PERMISSION

'Would that be OK?'
'I would normally ask for a chaperone because you will need to open or remove your shirt, but are you alright to continue?'
'Let me know if you are uncomfortable at any point.'
Whilst talking to the patient, look for features of anxiety or shortness of breath.

CLINICAL PROCEDURE

Remember: inspection, palpation, percussion and auscultation.
Ideally, the patient should be examined from their right and on an examination couch.

Hands:	sweaty, hot/cold, erythematous/cyanosed
	nails for splinter haemorrhages/clubbing
Radial pulse:	rate, rhythm, volume
Blood pressure:	with patient sitting, remove clothing from arm
JVP:	lie patient at 45 degrees and observe
Face:	look at face, eyes, tongue and mouth
Carotid pulse:	palpate for its character
Inspection:	inspect chest for any abnormalities, e.g. thoracotomy scar
	observe breathing pattern
Palpate:	feel for the apex beat and for any heaves or thrills
Auscultate:	listen to the heart sounds: try to pick up any added sounds and abnormal flow murmurs
	listen over the carotids

Lungs:	listen to the lungs for any effusions or signs of heart failure **percuss** over the lung fields for evidence of basal crepitations and reduced breath sounds
Abdominal aorta:	if time allows, examine the abdomen for evidence of aortic aneurysm
Other pulses:	femoral, popliteal, anterior tibial and dorsalis pedis (if concerned about peripheral vascular disease)
Oedema:	ankle for pitting oedema; if present, how extensive?

THANK THE PATIENT

FOR EXTRA MARKS

Heart auscultation: apex (mitral area)
lower left sternal edge
right and left of the manubrium (aortic and pulmonary areas)

Whilst examining the patient, ask about their medical history, in particular smoking, hypertension, diabetes, cholesterol and family history of heart disease.

Explain that, ideally, you'd like to take the patient for a walk to test their exercise tolerance.

Test the urine (haematuria in endocarditis).

Eyes (hypertensive retinopathy).

JVP is elevated if the top is 4 cm above the sternal angle.

Causes of raised JVP: congestive cardiac failure
tricuspid regurgitation
pulmonary embolism
tamponade.

STATION 4: PANIC DISORDER

THE EXAMINER'S MARK SHEET	
Communication	Simple management approach
Empathy	Answering other questions
Diagnosis	Global rating

INTRODUCE YOURSELF

'Hello, nice to meet you. My name is Dr Smith.'

SET THE SCENE

'I've been told you've been having panic attacks. Is this correct?
'Has anyone spoken to you about a diagnosis based on your anxiety symptoms?'

ASK PERMISSION

'Would it be OK to ask you about the anxiety attacks?'
Find out more details about the episodes.
Let the examiner know you are considering the diagnosis by going through the
diagnostic criteria for the anxiety disorders associated with panic.

TAKE A HISTORY OF PANIC: KEY AREAS

Panic disorder:

At least several attacks per month
Panic attacks in the absence of objective danger
Unpredictable
Free from anxiety between attacks

Differential diagnosis

Other anxiety/neurotic disorder, e.g. social phobia can lead to panic, such as
speaking to a group of people.
Depressive disorders lead to anxiety and sometimes panic.
Organic or physical disease must be ruled out, e.g. hyperthyroidism.

The presence of panic attacks does not necessarily mean this represents panic
disorder. For a diagnosis of panic disorder, several unpredictable and unprovoked
attacks should occur within a month.

MANAGEMENT
Psychological
CBT: cognitive restructuring and exposure techniques.
Training in anxiety management: breathing control and relaxation training.
Ongoing assessment and education about the nature of the disorder and the role of hyperventilation (common fears of those who panic and the fight and flight response).
Try not to avoid any of the feared situations, as this may lead to reinforcement of the learned fear response and agoraphobia may develop.

Medication
SSRIs
Some TCAs, e.g. clomipramine

ASK WHETHER SHE HAS ANY QUESTIONS

THANK HER

FOR EXTRA MARKS
Cognitive therapy is useful for treating the fears seen in panic disorder.
Fear of losing control: it is helpful to tell the patient that there is no documented report of anyone losing control and dying in the context of a panic attack.

FURTHER READING
Know the features of panic disorder from ICD-10.

STATION 5: PARIETAL LOBE ASSESSMENT

THE EXAMINER'S MARK SHEET

Communication/rapport	Bilateral testing
Dominant lobe	Answering any questions
Non-dominant lobe	Global rating

INTRODUCE YOURSELF

'Hello, nice to meet you. My name is Dr Smith.'

SET THE SCENE

Explain what your role is and that his GP has asked you to see him.

ASK FOR PERMISSION

Ask him whether it would be OK if you went through some questions and tests that you ask everyone you see.
'Some of the things I'll be asking will be quite difficult, while others will be easier, but try not to worry if you make some mistakes.'
'Let me know if you are uncomfortable at any point or getting too tired.'

CLINICAL PROCEDURE: TEST THE FOLLOWING

Dominant parietal lobe function

Receptive dysphasia:	obvious from conversation.
Gerstmann's syndrome:	Finger agnosia: 'Point to left ring finger with right index finger.'
	Dyscalculia: simple arithmetic.
	Right–left disorientation: 'Touch left ear with right hand.'
	Agraphia: ask the patient to draw something.

Non-dominant parietal lobe function

Neglect (inattention):	neglects one side – ask him to draw a clock face with dials and numbers.
Prosopagnosia:	failure to recognise faces, e.g. Queen Elizabeth on a £5 note.
Anosognosia:	failure to recognise a disabled body part.
Constructional apraxia:	unable to copy visually presented drawing – ask him to copy interlocking pentagons.
Topographical disorientation:	difficult finding way, especially in new environment – ask whether he gets confused or lost in new places.

Bilateral lobe function

Astereognosia: inability to identify object through touch alone – ask him to identify, with his eyes closed, a key or coin.

Agraphagnosia: failure to identify letters drawn on the palm – ask him to identify, with his eyes closed, H or W drawn with the top of a pen on his palm.

THANK THE PATIENT

FOR EXTRA MARKS

Potential neurological consequences of parietal lobe damage include:

Homonymous lower quadrantanopia (optic radiation)
Astereognosis, reduced discrimination (sensory cortex)

STATION 6: INTOXICATED PATIENT

THE EXAMINER'S MARK SHEET	
Communication	Mental state assessment
Empathy	Answering other questions
History of events	Global rating

INTRODUCE YOURSELF

'Hello, my name's Dr Smith. I'm one of the psychiatrists.'

SET THE SCENE

'How are you feeling?'
'You've spent most of the night in A&E. You must be tired.'
'I wanted to ask you what happened this morning.'

ASK FOR PERMISSION

'Would that be OK?'
This is a scenario many have encountered in clinical practice. It is difficult, as specific tasks have not been set and the patient may not be entirely co-operative. Keep it *simple* and *safe*. Always consider *risk*. Speak slowly and clearly.
If you feel that he is too drunk or confused to assess, then you must do a cognitive assessment (this will probably take up all the time).

TAKE A HISTORY: KEY AREAS

History examples – you may have others to add:

Notice whether he appears dishevelled or well-dressed (he may be homeless).
What were the events that led up to his presentation?
Can he remember anything before coming to hospital?
How much did he have to drink?
Does he drink often, or was this a one-off?
Did he hurt himself at all/or get into a brawl (were the police involved)?
Has he taken anything else apart from alcohol (drugs/illicit substances)?
Does he live alone? Is there anyone we can contact to speak to about him?
Does he have any children?
Is anyone else involved in his care, such as a nurse, social worker or psychiatrist?
How has he been feeling in his mood?
Enquire about suicidality and possible overdose (the medics may not have taken paracetamol or salicylate levels).
Wish to harm others?

Assess his thoughts.
Enquire about psychotic phenomena.
Does he have insight?

Be prepared for issues of admission to arise if he claims to be suicidal.
Avoid negative statements and questions, even if he's difficult with you. Use encouraging and positive statements:
'I know it's hard at the moment, but I'd really appreciate it if you could answer some of my questions.'

ASK WHETHER HE HAS ANY QUESTIONS

THANK HIM

FOR EXTRA MARKS

This OSCE station assesses your ability to control difficult situations. It is an exercise in getting as much information from the patient as possible in a sensitive manner. Pay attention to risk issues.

In reality, the following would need to be excluded: trauma, hypoglycaemia, hypothermia, hepatic encephalopathy, sepsis, electrolyte abnormalities and alcohol withdrawal.

FURTHER READING

Simpson M, Buckman R, Stewart M, *et al.* Doctor–patient communication: the Toronto consensus statement. *Br Med J* 1991; 303: 1385–7.

STATION 7: PSYCHOSIS

THE EXAMINER'S MARK SHEET	
Communication	Eliciting psychosis
Empathy	Answering other questions
Mental state	Global rating

INTRODUCE YOURSELF

'Hello, nice to meet you. My name is Dr Smith.'

SET THE SCENE

'I wanted to talk to you about how you have been feeling recently.'

ASK FOR PERMISSION

'Would that be OK?'
Use open questions to start:
'Has anything been worrying you?'
'Why did you turn yourself in to the police?'

MENTAL STATE EXAMINATION: KEY AREAS

Cover all the areas of mental state examination, but don't feel you have to follow a strict order. The skilful clinician will allow the interview to flow.

Appearance and behaviour:	dishevelled/unkempt, movement disorder (catatonia), restlessness (EPSE), rapport, eye contact
Speech:	rate, rhythm, volume
Mood:	subjective and objective affect (?flat, anhedonic) somatic features self-esteem, guilt *suicide: ideation and intent*
Thoughts:	form, e.g. derailment, loosening of associations, flight of ideas, incoherence (word salad: 'knight's move thinking'), neologisms content: what he is actually thinking (delusions, overvalued ideas, passivity, etc.)
Perceptions:	auditory, visual, olfactory, gustatory, tactile hallucinations mood congruence?
Cognitive state:	MMSE (abbreviated if there is only a little time)

Insight:	his concept of what is happening
	is it due to mental illness?
	'Do/could medicines help you?'
	'Would you take medication to help?' (adherence)

ASK WHETHER HE HAS ANY QUESTIONS

THANK HIM

FOR EXTRA MARKS

Direct your questioning in the MSE according to the case, as time is limited. This patient is likely to be psychotic, so ask the relevant questions.

Know your diagnostic criteria for schizophrenia, according to ICD-10:

A. Passivity of thought
B. Delusions of control/passivity, delusional perception
C. Auditory hallucinations; running commentary, third person
D. Delusions (persistent) of other kinds, culturally inappropriate and impossible, e.g. political identity or superhuman abilities
E. Persistent hallucinations in any modality
F Breaks in train of thought
G. Catatonic behaviour (excitement, posturing, waxy flexibility, negativism, mutism, stupor)
H. Negative symptoms (significant and consistent change in the overall quality of some aspects of personal behaviour, manifest as loss of interest, aimlessness, social withdrawal)

Diagnosis usually requires one clear symptom from A–D, or two or more from E–H, present for most of the time for 1 month or more.

OTHER LIKELY 'PSYCHOSIS' OSCES

This young man has been taken to the A&E department having been breaking things up in his apartment. Elicit psychotic symptoms.

This bus driver is saying strange things. Both family and work colleagues have become concerned. The police have been called after he threatened someone who complained that his work is suffering. Examine his mental state.

STATION 8: CHRONIC FATIGUE SYNDROME (NEURASTHENIA)

THE EXAMINER'S MARK SHEET	
Communication	Simple treatment advice
Empathy	Answering other questions
Diagnosis discussion	Global rating

INTRODUCE YOURSELF

'Hello, nice to meet you. My name is Dr Smith.'

SET THE SCENE

'I wanted to talk to you about your illness and the impact it's had on you.'
'Has anyone spoken to you about a diagnosis based on your symptoms?'

ASK PERMISSION

'Would it be OK to ask you about your current symptoms?'
Work through her current symptoms and history of events to clarify the diagnosis. Let the examiner know that you are considering the diagnosis by going through the diagnostic criteria.

TAKE A HISTORY OF CHRONIC FATIGUE SYNDROME: KEY AREAS

From the case history, the most likely diagnosis is chronic fatigue syndrome (CFS), a debilitating and complex disorder characterized by profound fatigue, not improved by bed-rest and often exacerbated by physical or mental activity. Functioning is at a substantially lower level of activity than before the illness.

DIAGNOSTIC FEATURES

Patients have severe chronic fatigue for 6 months or longer, other medical conditions having been excluded.
Concurrently, four or more of the following symptoms are present:

Substantial impairment in short-term memory or concentration
Sore throat
Tender lymph nodes
Muscle pain
Multi-joint pain without swelling or redness
Headaches of a new type
Unrefreshing sleep
Post-exertional malaise lasting more than 24 hours

The symptoms must have persisted or recurred during at least 6 months of illness and must not have predated the fatigue.

Patients often reject a psychiatric aetiology, so be careful not to antagonise the individual. Don't get into a battle of trying to label her with something that she refuses to accept. One approach might be:

'I can see you're not happy with the suggestion of chronic fatigue syndrome. May I ask why?'

'That's just my opinion. I'm sorry to upset you. Can I talk through with you why I think it might be chronic fatigue syndrome?'

TREATMENT APPROACH

Graded physical activity, but crucially avoid increasing the level of fatigue – avoid push–crash phenomenon

Family education

CBT

Pharmacology: due to sensitivity, begin with very low doses and increase slowly; antidepressants are of use in some individuals

ASK WHETHER SHE HAS ANY QUESTIONS

THANK HER

FOR EXTRA MARKS

Know the ICD-10 criteria for neurasthenia.

In some cases, CFS can persist for years. The cause or causes of CFS have not been identified and no specific diagnostic tests are available.

Care must be taken to exclude other known and often treatable conditions before a diagnosis of CFS is made.

DIFFERENTIAL DIAGNOSIS

Fibromyalgia
Chronic mononucleosis

Chronic fatigue is commonly associated with these.

TREATABLE ILLNESSES THAT CAN RESULT IN FATIGUE

Hypothyroidism
Sleep apnoea, narcolepsy
Depressive disorders
Mononucleosis
Eating disorders
Cancer
Autoimmune disease
Hormonal disorders
Subacute infections
Diabetes

FURTHER READING

Fischler B. Review of clinical and psychobiological dimensions of the chronic fatigue syndrome: differentiation from depression and contribution of sleep dysfunctions. *Sleep Med Rev* 1999; 3: 131–46.

STATION 9: TESTAMENTARY CAPACITY

THE EXAMINER'S MARK SHEET	
Communication	Relevant mental state examination
Empathy	Answering other questions
Testamentary capacity	Global rating

INTRODUCE YOURSELF

'Hello, nice to meet you. My name is Dr Smith.'

SET THE SCENE

'Have you had any concerns about your memory recently?'
'I understand you've recently completed a will. Is that right?'
'I have been asked to see you today because sometimes memory problems can affect one's ability to construct an appropriate will.'

ASK FOR PERMISSION

'Would you be happy to talk to me about this?'

ASSESS TESTAMENTARY CAPACITY: KEY AREAS

Usually, you need to explain who has requested the assessment and why. Ordinarily, all relevant medical and psychiatric records, and also an estimate of the value and nature of the estate, would be available.

The specific components of capacity can be assessed by asking about her understanding of a will and its purpose. A general estimate of her property and its value is critical. Ask about the potential heirs and her wishes with respect to each. Reasons to include or exclude individuals should be explored. Requirements for testamentary capacity:

The person must know that they are making a will.
The person must know the nature and extent of their property.
The person must know the legal heirs.
The person must know the manner in which the will distributes the property.

Clinical history and MMSE are very important.
A number of conditions can interfere with valid will completion. Major psychiatric illnesses, such as schizophrenia and dementia, are common examples. Their presence, however, does not always mean that the individual lacks testamentary capacity. Someone with a psychotic illness who believes that the FBI has bugged their apartment because they can communicate with aliens may know very well the size of their estate, their children and how it should be divided between them.

In assessing testamentary capacity in this case, the following should be determined:

Is or was there a major psychiatric disorder?
Does this psychiatric disorder impair the ability to know she was making a will?
Does this disorder impair her ability to know the nature and value of the estate?
Does this disorder impair her ability to identify the heirs that would usually be considered?
Are delusions present that involve the estate or heirs?
Is the individual vulnerable to undue influence?

ASK WHETHER SHE HAS ANY QUESTIONS

THANK HER

FOR EXTRA MARKS

Testamentary capacity is the ability to execute a valid will.
Psychosis/delusions that would invalidate a person's capacity to make a will often involve their heirs in a negative way.
Elderly people are often advised by lawyers to have an evaluation of testamentary capacity at the time the will is executed.
Videotaping is used increasingly at the time of will execution, which can later be used in court.

FURTHER READING

Arie T. Some legal aspects of mental capacity. *Br Med J* 1996; 313: 156–8.

STATION 10: TRAVEL AND LITHIUM

THE EXAMINER'S MARK SHEET	
Communication	Travel and destination
Empathy	Answering other questions
Before the trip	Global rating

INTRODUCE YOURSELF

'Hello, nice to meet you. My name is Dr Smith.'

SET THE SCENE

'I'm pleased to hear you're having a holiday, but there are some important things to consider because of the lithium.'

FIND OUT WHAT THEY ALREADY KNOW

'Have you been away on lithium before?'
'What do you already know about travelling whilst taking lithium?'

INFORMATION ON LITHIUM
Before the trip

Travelling means an extra risk in BPAD, due mainly to transitions, instability and physical demands.
Ensure that travel plans are discussed between doctor and patient:
'Before long-distance travel, it is best that you reduce as many unnecessary activities as possible and do only the essentials.'
'Travel can cause a lot of stress due to excitement before leaving, the physical stress of flying and changes in the environment. It is important that you keep to your routine in the days leading up to your trip.'
Anticipation and excitement can cause insomnia. Short-term benzodiazepines may be used in the days before travel. Also, practising relaxation techniques before bed can help.

Provide a medical declaration

Explain that you will give them a report to take, should they need medical assistance at any point. This should state:

Name, date of birth, diagnosis, and the name and contact details of the hospital the patient attends for regular treatment
List of all medications
Lithium: dosage, treatment per day, brand name
Last recorded lithium blood level

Travelling and destination

Jet lag can precipitate mood fluctuations, so a short-acting benzodiazepine can be useful. It is important to keep well-hydrated during the flight, and it is a good idea to avoid alcohol. Sleeping tablets for the purposes of the flight can also help.

Any cause of fluid disturbance, such as vomiting, diarrhoea and excessive perspiration, may precipitate lithium toxicity. Therefore, especially in hot environments, it is important to take adequate fluids and salts. It is useful to pack remedies for common gastrointestinal upset and fever.

Travel insurance including health cover is vital.

ASK WHETHER THEY HAVE ANY QUESTIONS

THANK THEM

FOR EXTRA MARKS

Prepare for the worst! Anything that causes stress, such as stolen luggage or cancelled flights, potentially can lead to mood disturbance. Split the medication between suitcases and hand luggage (or a companion's luggage). Take extra supplies of medication in case flights are delayed/cancelled. Remind the patient to take their lithium card, which will remind them of the signs of lithium toxicity.

If they intend to travel alone, then they should consider wearing a medical alert bracelet.

FURTHER READING

Kleindienst N, Greil W. Lithium in the long-term treatment of bipolar disorders. *Eur Arch Psychiatry Clin Neurosci* 2003; 253: 120–25.

STATION 11: X-RAY INTERPRETATION

THE EXAMINER'S MARK SHEET

Communication	Presentation of findings
Checking and orientating	Answering other questions
Film examination	Global rating

(The film shown below is normal.)

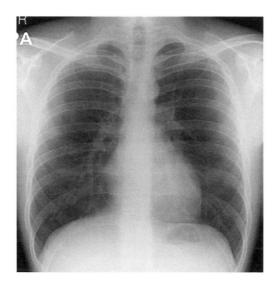

INTRODUCE YOURSELF

You do not need to introduce yourself in this scenario as your consultant will know you. You might have to present your findings in person or over the telephone. Be professional. Avoid lay terms.

SET THE SCENE

'This is Mr Stanley's chest radiograph. As you know, he's due ECT in a few days' time.'

COMMENT ON THE FILM

Be as systematic as possible.

Check that the radiograph is:

Named
Dated
Orientated correctly
Marked as AP (anteroposterior), PA (posteroanterior), supine or erect

Check X-ray *penetration*: vertebral bodies should just be seen through the heart on a chest radiograph.
Check for *rotation:* in the chest X-ray, look at the comparative size of the clavicles – they should be equal.
Comment on any *obvious abnormalities*, e.g. a mass. Comment on possible differential diagnoses if abnormal.

Look systematically at main structures:

Trachea:	should be central, slight inferior deviation to the right can be normal
Heart:	enlargement (cardiothoracic ratio is normally < 50 per cent)
Mediastinum:	aortic arch, lymph nodes, any shift
	hila, change in density, lymph nodes
Lungs:	pneumothorax
	bullous changes
	consolidation
	lesions/tumours
Diaphragm:	costophrenic angles should be sharp and clear
	right hemidiaphragm is usually slightly higher
	obvious gastric bubble
Soft tissues:	e.g. breast tissue
Bones:	vertebrae, clavicles, ribs

Summarise your findings.
Explain that the film will be reported on formally by one of the radiologists.

FOR EXTRA MARKS

You should talk through the above so that the examiner knows you are being systematic.
Comment on the 'radiograph' or 'film' rather than the 'X-ray'.
Bone causes much higher X-ray absorption, because of the high atomic weight of calcium.
Gas, fat and water are readily differentiated because of their different densities.
Don't rely solely on the X-ray for diagnosis. You would also want to examine the patient.

STATION 12: EROTOMANIA

THE EXAMINER'S MARK SHEET	
Communication	Risk
Clinical features	Answering other questions
Relevant mental state	Global rating

INTRODUCE YOURSELF

'Hello, nice to meet you. My name is Dr Smith.'

SET THE SCENE

'I was hoping to talk to you about how you've been feeling recently.'

ASK FOR PERMISSION

'Would that be OK?'

TAKE A HISTORY OF EROTOMANIA: KEY AREAS

'Your GP seems to have upset you at your last meeting. Do you remember what happened?'

Try to elicit the clinical features

In this case, the object of love is of *higher status*, is famous and has wealth. The object of love is *inaccessible*.

There may be a distinct time/event when the patient became convinced of the 'special relationship'. This may have been a brief meeting or sighting, e.g. at a pop concert.

A typical history will include that the *love object initiated the relationship*, that the patient communicates with him via covert mechanisms, and that there are messages from him in everyday life for her, e.g. on television.

Enquire about *stalking behaviour*. Often, a person with erotomania follows the person relentlessly and attempts to make contact by various means.

This may be an isolated delusional disorder or secondary to other conditions, particularly schizophrenia and mania.

A relevant MSE is important. There is usually an absence of hallucinations and no cognitive impairment.

Risk

It is important to ask about:

Any stalking behaviour now or in the past
Previous offences/trouble with the police

Feelings of aggression towards the love object or others
Previous love objects/relationships (any aggression?)

ASK WHETHER SHE HAS ANY QUESTIONS

THANK HER

FOR EXTRA MARKS

More common in women than men.

Often a chronic disorder.

To gain top marks, it is necessary to get a clear picture of the delusionary system, which can be intricate. There may be evidence of a complex set of beliefs around the perceived relationship. Try to get as much information as possible.

Another form of presentation includes the 'local' woman who becomes fixated on a 'local' man. In this case, the woman can become aggressive towards the man's wife or others whom she believes to be 'in the way'.

FURTHER READING

Segal JH. Erotomania revisited: from Kraepelin to DSM-III-R. *Am J Psychiatry* 1989; **146**: 1261–6.

EXAM 6

STATION 1

A GP has been put through to you on the telephone. He has just seen a patient with a 5-year history of bipolar affective disorder. She has remained very well for approximately 2 years, having required an admission 3 years ago when she was manic, psychotic and neglecting her own self-care. She has been taking an antidepressant and a mood stabiliser for the past 18 months. She does not take lithium.

She has been in a stable relationship with her boyfriend for 6 years and they would like to start a family. It is important for her to be able to breastfeed. The GP tells you that she asked about her medication and whether she should stop it before trying to conceive.

The GP asks your advice with regard to these issues.

[advice on page 168]

STATION 2

This man is self-presenting to drug services for the first time following a 3-year history of opiate misuse. He is noticed to be aggressive.

He wants to know how you can help him.

[advice on page 171]

STATION 3

A 72-year-old woman has been brought to A&E. She has become increasingly confused. She has a history of bipolar affective disorder, but no other details are available. She was able to tell the paramedics that her doctor had recently prescribed her a 'blood-pressure tablet'. The medical senior house officer has faxed you some results and asks for your opinion.

What are the abnormal findings?
What is the likely aetiology for this presentation?
What other investigations would you recommend?

Test	Result	Units	Reference range
Glucose	5.6	mmol/L	
TSH	2.86	mU/L	0.3–5.5
Vitamin B12	312	ng/L	180–1100
Folate	5.4	ug/L	3.0–13.0
Vitamin B12/folate/ferritin	27	ug/L	20–200
WBC	9	10^9/L	4–11
RBC	5.1	10^{12}/L	3.8–5.8
Hb	13.2	g/dL	11.5–15.5
PCV	0.47	L/L	0.37–0.47
MCV	80	fl	79–96
PLT	176	10^9/L	150–450
Na	132	mmol/L	135–145
K	3.2	mmol/L	3.5–5.0
Creat	102	umol/L	45–120
Ca	2.32	mmol/L	2.20–2.60
Phosph	1.10	mmol/L	0.80–1.40
Corr Ca	2.32	mmol/L	
T Prot	63	g/L	60–80
Albumin	43	g/L	35–50
T Bil	5	umol/L	3–20
Alk Phosph	94	u/L	30–130
AST	30	u/L	10–50
GGT	45	u/L	1–55

Urine dipstick	Mild protein
Microscopy	**Epithelial cells**

[advice on page 173]

STATION 4

This 24-year-old man has been a heavy user of cannabis for the past 6 years. His parents have noticed that he has become more withdrawn and feel his behaviour can be 'strange'. He has not been able to find work and spends much of his time smoking and listening to music.

Assess his mental state and explain the risks associated with cannabis.

[advice on page 175]

STATION 5

This patient is due his depot medication. There is no one else available to give it to him.

Give him his IM depot medication.

[advice on page 177]

STATION 6

Mr Thompson, a 32-year-old married accountant, has become increasingly preoccupied with personal cleanliness and orderliness in his house. He has been late for work persistently, delayed by a need to check that his appliances have been unplugged. You are the first psychiatric professional to see him.

Assess him for obsessions.
He wants to know whether he will get better.

[advice on page 180]

STATION 7

This patient has collapsed on the ward.

Perform a neurological examination of his lower limbs.

[advice on page 182]

STATION 8

Assess suicidal ideation in this gentleman, who was persuaded by his friend to attend the A&E department after hearing him speaking about wanting to die.

[advice on page 185]

STATION 9

You are the most senior psychiatrist on site. A more junior colleague has phoned you for some advice. He has just seen a 27-year-old man on the ward who is extremely agitated and seems to be disturbed by auditory hallucinations. He has pulled the fire extinguisher from the wall and has been smashing windows and attempting to injure staff and patients. The emergency team was called and has him in restraint. He has a diagnosis of schizophrenia and is already prescribed risperidone.

What advice will you give to your junior colleague?

[advice on page 187]

STATION 10

This woman has been referred to your clinic having asked her family doctor if she could see a psychiatrist. She reports tiredness and low mood in winter over the past few years.

She wants to know whether she has seasonal affective disorder.

[advice on page 190]

STATION 11

You are seeing an 81-year-old woman on the ward. She has not been coping at home. An MRI scan shows small-vessel disease and evidence of an ischaemic region in the left temporal area, probably an old cerebrovascular accident (CVA). As part of your cognitive assessment, you wish to consider her temporal lobe function.

Assess her temporal lobe function.

[advice on page 192]

STATION 12

This woman attends the community clinic wanting to speak to her husband's psychiatrist. She is angry that their sex life has deteriorated as a result of him taking an SSRI antidepressant.

Speak to this woman.

[advice on page 194]

STATION 1: PREGNANCY AND BREASTFEEDING

THE EXAMINER'S MARK SHEET	
Communication	Breastfeeding
Safety/risk issues	Answering other questions
Pregnancy	Global rating

INTRODUCE YOURSELF

'Hello, my name's Dr Smith.'
Remember to avoid lay terminology in this station.

SET THE SCENE

'Thank you for calling. This is a common problem for young women who are considering starting a family.'
Explain that you will try to help as much as possible, but that in the interests of safety you will be contacting the pharmacy drug information service in the hospital, or the nearest mother and baby unit team, for further advice.

FIND OUT WHAT THEY ALREADY KNOW

Ask the GP:

What drugs is the patient taking, and at what dosages?
Does the patient have any other children? If so, was she unwell at the time? What happened on that occasion?
Does she have any other relevant past medical history?

INFORMATION ON PREGNANCY AND BREASTFEEDING

The patient should be informed of the potential risks involved, in terms of relapsing illness, should she stop her medication, but she should also be informed of the potential risks to the fetus if she continues her medication. The patient should be commended for taking such a sensible approach in her preconception phase, but the decision to stop, change or continue medication should be a joint one between the medical team, the patient and her partner. Explain that, ideally, you would like to see the patient and also her medical records, but that the general advice is as follows:

Pregnancy

Antidepressant
TCAs are thought to be least harmful.
Neonatal withdrawal is possible if used in the last trimester.

SSRIs are also thought to be relatively safe but can be associated with neonatal discontinuation symptoms.

MAOIs should be avoided if possible.

If the patient has been very well for some time on a medication, then continuing may be the best all-round choice.

Medication given in the first trimester is associated with a higher percentage of malformations.

Mood stabiliser

Lithium should be avoided (not relevant here) due to risk of malformation.

Sodium valproate and carbamazepine are also linked to fetal malformations (spina bifida) and should try to be avoided.

Folate supplementation should be recommended, even if the above are not prescribed.

Consider stopping medication if long period of remission.

No mood stabilisers are thought to be entirely safe in pregnancy.

If she decides to stop the medication, then her team and GP should provide regular support and monitoring of her mental state throughout the pregnancy. If she continues with medication, then the fetus should undergo regular monitoring.

Breastfeeding

Little/no evidence base currently exists.

Antidepressant

Most TCAs enter breast milk in small amounts, but manufacturers advise avoidance (see *BNF*).

Most SSRIs enter the breast milk, and manufacturers suggest avoidance.

Mood stabiliser

Lithium has been reported to cause infant toxicity (not relevant here).

Small amounts of carbamazepine, valproate and lamotrigine are thought to pass into breast milk. The general advice would be not to breastfeed. If the mother does breastfeed, then the baby must be monitored for evidence of drug effects and toxicity.

ASK WHETHER HE HAS ANY OTHER QUESTIONS

THANK HIM

FOR EXTRA MARKS

ECT has been used with good effect in pregnancy.
Expressing and discarding milk from peak plasma times can help limit infant exposure.
Use the lowest therapeutic doses if continuing with medication.
Try to avoid drugs with long half-lives.
Try to take drugs once daily before the baby's longest sleep (usually at night), to avoid peak plasma levels.

FURTHER READING

Taylor D, Paton C, Kerwin R. *The South London and Maudsley NHS Trust 2003 Prescribing Guidelines*, 7th edn. London: Martin Dunitz, 2003.
British Medical Association, Royal Pharmaceutical Society of Great Britain. *British National Formulary*. London: BMJ Books and Pharmaceutical Press.
Dodd S, Berk M. The pharmacology of bipolar disorder during pregnancy and breastfeeding. *Expert Opin Drug Saf* 2004; 3: 221–9.

STATION 2: OPIATE ADDICTION

THE EXAMINER'S MARK SHEET	
Communication	Intervention strategies
Drug history	Answering other questions
Harm minimisation	Global rating

INTRODUCE YOURSELF

'Hello, nice to meet you. My name is Dr Smith.'

SET THE SCENE

'Thank you for coming here today.'
'Most people that come here have problems with drug addiction. Can I ask what's been happening in your case?'
An open question allows the patient to talk and may diffuse any anger.
Safety first! If he is angry, comment on it: 'Something seems to be upsetting you. What has happened?'
An empathetic, non-confrontational approach is best.

FIND OUT WHAT HE ALREADY KNOWS

'Do you know anything about strategies used to help people come off drugs?'
Why is this man presenting for treatment now?

INFORMATION ON OPIATE ADDICTION AND DETOXIFICATION

Before the commencement of any substitution therapy, confirm that opiates are indeed being taken. Urine drug testing is important to confirm this – mention towards the end if the patient is agitated. This prevents the possibility of an iatrogenic overdose. A brief history of current use should be taken.
Levels of *motivation* need to be ascertained by asking the patient to outline the benefits of continuing 'using' as opposed to stopping.
The majority of early intervention strategies are focused on returning to less hazardous means of drug-taking rather than total abstinence, i.e. the *harm-minimisation model* – use clean needles/syringes, safe injecting techniques, safe sex, health awareness (HIV, hepatitis C), maintain contact with addiction services. Depending on the severity of the addiction, this man may need inpatient detoxification or daily attendance at the addiction clinic.
The main objectives are to limit the damage that occurs during drug use, to limit the periods of drug use, and to prevent the likelihood of relapse.

Substitute prescribing

Treatment options include methadone maintenance and buprenorphine (opioid substitutes).

Advise about short-, medium- and long-term treatment options:

Short-term detoxification from opiates
Medium-term substitute therapy
Long-term rehabilitation and removal of substitute therapy

Psychological approaches

Substitute prescribing together with psychotherapy can be helpful for some users. Motivational interviewing and relapse prevention interventions are examples.

ASK WHETHER HE HAS ANY QUESTIONS

THANK HIM

FOR EXTRA MARKS

A rapid assessment of the man's previous history, current levels of motivation and a simple description of the treatment options are required to gain top marks. As there is a lot to cover, watch your time carefully.

FURTHER READING

Strang J, Marks I, Dawe S, *et al.* Type of hospital setting and treatment outcome with heroin addicts: results from a randomised trial. *Br J Psychiatry* 1997; 171: 335–9.

STATION 3: DATA INTERPRETATION

THE EXAMINER'S MARK SHEET	
Communication	Investigations
Abnormal findings	Answering other questions
Aetiology	Global rating

INTRODUCE YOURSELF

Remain professional when dealing with a colleague.

SET THE SCENE

'Thank you for sending the blood results.'
'This lady has become even more confused since she's attended hospital – is that right?'

FIND OUT WHAT THEY ALREADY KNOW

'We have no information at the moment other than these blood results – is that correct?'
'Have you excluded other causes of confusion, such as a head injury or CVA?'

DATA INTERPRETATION

You may be asked to interpret results as part of an OSCE. Take your time to look at the results properly before talking. It is unlikely to be very complicated, and most marks will be awarded for a logical approach.

Abnormal findings

Low sodium and potassium
Insignificant findings on urine microscopy
Otherwise unremarkable

Aetiology

This is an older adult with a history of BPAD and confusion, having been started on what sounds like an antihypertensive. No other information is available. A biological aetiology such as an infection needs to be considered, but it is very important to exclude lithium toxicity in this case. Thiazide diuretics prescribed for hypertension could present in this way in a lithium-treated patient. They induce a mild hyponatraemia and hypokalaemia; the kidneys respond by reabsorbing both sodium and lithium (which is treated renally as sodium), leading to reduced lithium clearance and subsequent toxicity.

Ask whether the patient has the clinical features of lithium toxicity:

Gastrointestinal: anorexia, nausea, diarrhoea
CNS: drowsiness, confusion, ataxia, muscle weakness, coarse tremor, muscle twitching, agitation
Severe toxicity: increased disorientation, seizures, coma, death

INVESTIGATIONS

Urgent lithium levels
Seek expert advice from poisons information centre

In serious toxicity (> 2.0 mmol/L), haemodialysis may be necessary. Otherwise, supportive measures, stop diuretics, encourage adequate fluid intake (oral/IV), correct electrolyte abnormalities, control convulsions if present. Frequent lithium levels (every 6–12 hours) to monitor progress.

ASK WHETHER THEY HAVE ANY OTHER QUESTIONS

THANK THEM

FOR EXTRA MARKS

Common causes of lithium toxicity:

Dehydration
Poor renal function
Infection
Diuretics/NSAIDs
Overdose

Therapeutic lithium levels 0.4–1.0 mmol/L.

FURTHER READING

Tyrer SP. Lithium intoxication: appropriate treatment. *CNS Drugs* 1996; 6: 426–39.

STATION 4: CANNABIS

THE EXAMINER'S MARK SHEET	
Communication	Answering other questions
Relevant mental state	Global rating
Cannabis risks	

INTRODUCE YOURSELF

'Hello, nice to meet you. My name is Dr Smith.'
The actor is likely to be disinterested in what you say. Be patient and nice to him! Don't become frustrated – it will show.

SET THE SCENE

'I'm one of the psychiatrists. I've been asked to see you'
'Your parents have some concerns about you. Do you know what they might be worried about?'
'I wanted to find out how you have been feeling recently.'

ASK FOR PERMISSION

'Would that be OK?'

MENTAL STATE EXAMINATION: KEY AREAS

In this case, you have to undertake a MSE focusing particularly on depressive and psychotic features (refer to OSCE Exam 5, Station 7): appearance and behaviour, speech, mood, thoughts, perceptions, cognitive state and insight.

CANNABIS RISKS

Ask about use of cannabis, other illicit drugs and alcohol. Get an idea of the quantities used and the costs involved.
Ask what the benefits are from smoking cannabis. Can he identify any associated risks?

Carcinoma: risk is at least as great as, if not greater than, that with tobacco. Chronic inflammatory and precancerous changes in the airways have been demonstrated in cannabis users. The increased risk of bronchial cancer is thought to be proportional to the amount of cannabis use.
Ischaemic heart disease.
Psychosis: the epidemiological association between cannabis use and schizophrenia most likely represents a causal role of cannabis in precipitating the onset or relapse of schizophrenia in susceptible individuals.

Depression: a weaker but significant link between cannabis and depression has been found in various cohort studies.

Paranoia.

Panic attacks.

Depersonalisation-derealisation.

Dependence: cannabis dependence, both behavioural and physical, is thought to occur in about seven to ten per cent of regular users; early onset of use, and in particular weekly or daily use, is a strong predictor of future dependence.

Cognitive impairment: cannabis use does affect short-term memory, the ability to concentrate and co-ordination. Longer-term effects are still unclear.

Some of these symptoms may become apparent during the MSE.

ASK WHETHER HE HAS ANY QUESTIONS

THANK HIM

FOR EXTRA MARKS

Cannabis contains more than 400 chemicals, the main one being delta-9-tetrahydrocannabinol.

On 29 January 2004, cannabis was reclassified from a class B to a class C drug in the UK. It is still a controlled drug, so production, supply and possession remain illegal.

In total, the evidence indicates that regular heavy use of cannabis carries significant risk for the individual user.

SUPPORT GROUPS

Recovery: www.recovery.org.uk – simple information and advice from an alcohol and drug site aimed at young people

Quit: www.quit.org.uk

FURTHER READING

Leweke FM, Gerth CW, Klosterkotter J. Cannabis-associated psychosis: current status of research. *CNS Drugs* 2004; 18: 895–910.

STATION 5: INTRAMUSCULAR INJECTION

THE EXAMINER'S MARK SHEET	
Communication	Injection technique
Patient consideration	Answering other questions
Explanation	Global rating

INTRODUCE YOURSELF

A mannequin is provided. Treat it with respect!
'Hello, nice to meet you. My name is Dr Smith.'

SET THE SCENE

Explain to the patient what you are about to do. Talk as you go along, so the examiner knows what you are doing.
'I was hoping to give you your injection today.'

ASK FOR PERMISSION

'Would that be OK?'
'I would normally ask for a chaperone, but are you alright to continue?'
'Let me know if you are uncomfortable at any point.'

CLINICAL PROCEDURE

Check that the depot is the correct drug and dose.
Ask for the drug card if it is not provided.
Check that the date on the vial has not expired.
Use a 20–25 G 1–3-inch needle.
A 3–5-ml syringe is needed.
Put on gloves.
Draw up the depot.
Explain to the patient that you are nearly ready.
Expose the buttock area and clean the upper outer quadrant on one side with an alcohol wipe. Clean from the centre outwards.
Tap the injection site gently to stimulate the nerve endings and reduce pain when the needle is injected.

Use the z-track technique (see below)

Tell the patient: 'You'll feel a sharp prick now.'
In the correct location* (see below) and at a 90-degree angle to the skin, quickly and firmly push the needle through and into the muscle. Before injecting the

medication, remember to pull back on the plunger to ensure that you are not in a blood vessel. Slowly inject the depot into the muscle.

Z-track injection

This method of IM injection prevents leakage or tracking of the drug into the subcutaneous tissue (SCT).

Place a finger on the skin surface at the injection site. With this finger, pull the skin and SCT out of alignment with the underlying muscle (half an inch).

Insert the needle at a 90-degree angle at the site where the finger was initially, inject the drug and withdraw the needle.

Finally, remove the finger and allow the skin and SCT to return their original positions. This method breaks the needle track through the different tissue layers, trapping the drug in the muscle.

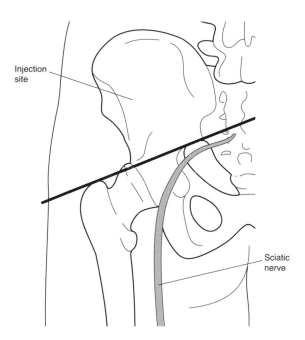

Injecting above an imaginary line between the posterior superior iliac spine and the greater trochanter of the femur (or in the upper outer quadrant) will avoid the sciatic nerve.

THANK THE PATIENT

FOR EXTRA MARKS

Ask whether it would be OK to inject in the buttock area, as some patients rotate sites.

An older patient may require a small pressure bandage afterwards, as reduced tissue elasticity makes bleeding/bruising more likely.

Other IM sites: deltoid, ventrogluteal, vastus lateralis.

IM injections should not be administered at inflamed, oedematous or irritated areas, moles, birthmarks or scar tissue.

Complications at depot injection site: infection, SCT irritation, abscess, tissue fibrosis.

FURTHER READING

Nicoll L, Hesby A. Intramuscular injection: an integrative research review and guideline for evidence-based practice. *Appl Nurs Res* 2002; **15**: 149–62.

STATION 6: OBSESSIONS: ASSESSMENT

THE EXAMINER'S MARK SHEET	
Communication	Prognosis
Empathy	Answering other questions
Obsessions: assessment	Global rating

INTRODUCE YOURSELF
'Hello, nice to meet you. My name is Dr Smith.'

SET THE SCENE
'I've heard there have been some difficulties recently. Can you tell me about them?' (open question).

ASK FOR PERMISSION
'Would that be OK?'

TAKE A HISTORY OF OBSESSIONS: KEY AREAS
Obsessional thoughts can be experienced as ideas, mental images or impulses to act. Always consider *risk* and enquire about thoughts to harm themselves or others.

Obsessions
'Have you noticed that you have to keep checking things that you have checked moments before?' (Examples might include electrical appliances, door-handles and taps.)
'What happens if you try to stop yourself from doing this?'
'What about touching or counting things?'
'Some people we see spend a lot of time trying to keep clean, like washing their hands repeatedly. Do you ever find yourself doing this?'
'Why do you think you do this?' (Contamination?)
'How would you feel if you were prevented from hand-washing?'
'Do you have any other similar behaviours that have to be done in a particular way?'
'Do you have thoughts that keep coming into your mind that you find difficult to stop?' (Obsessional thoughts.)
'Are they there all the time?' (Unpleasantly repetitive?)
Are they upsetting?' (Nearly always distressing for the patient.)
'Are you able to stop them?' (Resisted, unsuccessfully?)
'How do you stop them?'
'Are they your own thoughts?' (Testing for passivity.)
'How has this affected your life?'

PROGNOSIS

Ask whether anyone has discussed a diagnosis with him.
If not, explain briefly what you think the diagnosis is (has he heard of OCD?).
Prognosis varies:

Seventy per cent of 'mild' cases improve after 1–5 years.
Thirty-three per cent of severe (hospital-admitted) patients improve after
1–5 years.
The longer the duration of the illness, the worse the prognosis.
A need for symmetry is associated with poor prognosis in males.
More likely to be chronic in the absence of significant depressive features.

Be honest, but also instil some hope when appropriate to do so.

ASK WHETHER HE HAS ANY OTHER QUESTIONS

THANK HIM

FOR EXTRA MARKS

Obsessional thoughts and compulsive acts often occur together. The patient
may find it difficult to separate them. Don't worry if the patient starts talking
about compulsive acts – it will build a better picture. However, make sure you
cover the obsessional component fully.
Obsessional symptoms may be part of another underlying disorder, e.g.
depressive illness (20 per cent), schizophrenia, early dementia and other
organic brain syndromes, anorexia nervosa, generalised anxiety state.

If asked about onset: 65 per cent before age 25 years
                        15 per cent after age 35 years

STATION 7: LOWER-LIMB EXAMINATION

THE EXAMINER'S MARK SHEET	
Communication	Sensation
Inspection/tone	Reflexes
Power	Global rating

INTRODUCE YOURSELF

'Hello, nice to meet you. My name is Dr Smith.'

EXPLAIN WHAT YOU HAVE BEEN ASKED TO DO

'I'm sorry to hear about your collapse on the ward. Are you feeling OK now?'
'I would like to examine your legs.'

ASK FOR PERMISSION

'Would that be OK?'
'Let me know if you are uncomfortable at any point.'

CLINICAL PROCEDURE

The subject should, ideally, be on an examination couch.
Examine from the patient's right-hand side.
By explaining what you are doing at each step, you are letting the examiner know that you are competent.

Inspection

Look for any obvious abnormalities/deformities
Skin colour/rashes
Muscle wasting
Muscle fasciculation (motor neuron disease)
Restlessness (EPSE)

Tone

Examine each leg by moving it passively at the hip and knee joints. Roll the leg sideways, backwards and forwards on the couch/bed. Lift the knee and let it drop. With the legs hanging over the side of the bed, lift the leg and let it drop. Observe natural swing at the knee.
Look in particular for increase/decrease in tone and evidence of cogwheeling or lead-pipe rigidity.

Power

Ask the subject to:

Lift his leg up from the hip – 'Don't let me push it down.'
Bend his knee – 'Don't let me straighten your leg.'
Keep his knee bent – 'Push your leg against my hand.'
Point his toes up towards his face – 'Don't let me push them down.'

Remember to do both sides and compare findings.

Co-ordination

Ask the subject to place his heel just below his knee, run it down his shin and then back up and down once more. Ask him to repeat with the other foot.

Reflexes

Knee jerk
Ankle jerk
Plantar response

Sensation

Ideally, one should test light touch (cotton-wool) and pinprick in the following areas (although, for the purposes of the exam, a finger touch should suffice):

Outer thigh (L2)
Inner thigh (L3)
Inner calf (L4)
Outer calf (L5)
Inner foot (L5)
Outer foot (S1)

Ask the subject to close his eyes and tell you when he feels something. Compare sensation in both legs, i.e. don't do one leg completely and then move to the next. Reassure him that you will be gentle.
Vibration sense can be tested in the big toe (if a tuning fork is present), as can joint position sense (up and down).

Gait

Ask the subject whether he can walk for you
Observe his normal gait
Then ask him to walk heel to toe (ataxia)

Romberg's test

Feet together arms outstretched, closed eyes
Take care to ensure he does not fall

THANK HIM

FOR EXTRA MARKS

Romberg's test is positive only if the subject is more unsteady with eyes closed.

A positive Romberg's test indicates a loss of proprioception, e.g. subacute combined degeneration of the cord, tabes dorsalis.

STATION 8: RISK ASSESSMENT: SUICIDAL PATIENT

THE EXAMINER'S MARK SHEET	
Communication skills	Risk assessment
Empathy	Answering other questions
Thoughts of self-harm/plans	Global rating

INTRODUCE YOURSELF

'Hello, nice to meet you. My name is Dr Smith.'

SET THE SCENE

'I wanted to talk to you about how you've been feeling in yourself recently.'

ASK FOR PERMISSION

'Would that be OK?'

'Has anything been worrying you?'

TAKE A HISTORY OF SUICIDAL IDEATION: KEY AREAS

Start by assessing mood

A good way to lead into personal questions in this case is to ask about mood. He may be severely depressed and on the verge of attempting to kill himself.

Then ask about thoughts of self-harm

'I am sorry to hear you have not been feeling well over the past weeks. Sometimes, when we become low in mood, thoughts of harming oneself can creep in. Has this happened to you at all?'

Ask about intention to self-harm

'That must be very difficult. Can I ask whether you have ever thought about acting on these thoughts? Do you have specific plans to harm yourself? What do they involve?'

Ask about death wish

'Sometimes, one can feel as if they would be better off dead. Has this been the case?'

Assess the seriousness of the death wish

Explore sensitively why the man wants to be dead. Ask about previous attendances and attempts or self-harm.

Precipitant/change in mental state

Ask about any recent events or stressors that may have affected his mental state.

Risk assessment

Should cover the following:

Use of alcohol/drugs
Unemployment
Single/widowed/divorced (interpersonal difficulties)
Children
Risk to others
Command hallucinations
His view on any intervention or DSH
Any supportive relationships
Compliance with previous interventions, services, etc.
Presence of chronic/painful illness

ASK WHETHER HE HAS ANY QUESTIONS

THANK HIM

FOR EXTRA MARKS

Risk issues are always examined in one form or another. Delivering a
polished performance at such a station is important, as your competitors will
have this station covered. The good marks will go to those who appear the
most competent and understanding. This comes with practice.

Risk issues are also considered in Exam 1, Station 12, and Exam 8, Stations 8
and 9.

STATION 9: RAPID TRANQUILISATION

THE EXAMINER'S MARK SHEET	
Communication	Rapid tranquilisation
Junior support	Risk/safety
General advice	Global rating

INTRODUCE YOURSELF

'Hello, this is Dr Smith speaking.'

SET THE SCENE

'It sounds like things are quite difficult. Would you like me to come over and help, or are you OK?'

Do what you would normally do in such situations: be safe, be sensible and take senior advice when needed.

FIND OUT WHAT THEY ALREADY KNOW

'The patient is currently in restraint. Is the situation stable?'

The prime concern is for the safety of the individual involved, the other patients and the staff. If the situation is becoming unmanageable, then the police or hospital security should be called for support.

Advise your colleague to talk to the nursing staff and look through the patient's medical notes. Look for any known drug allergies and current and previous medications. Are there any other reasons for his agitation (organic, illicit drugs)? Offer to assist your colleague if he is inexperienced.

INFORMATION ON RAPID TRANQUILISATION

Let the junior psychiatrist (and, more importantly, the examiner) know that this is a psychiatric emergency and he should be considering rapid tranquilisation (RT). RT should be considered only when other methods of de-escalation have failed. These include psychological and behavioural approaches. Offering the patient PRN medication may also eliminate the need for RT.

According to the *South London and Maudsley NHS Trust 2003 Prescribing Guidelines*, the following steps should be considered (you should not be expected to know doses – if pressed, say you would refer to the *BNF*/pharmacy/senior colleague):

1. Try to de-escalate the situation (e.g. time out, placement).
2. Offer oral medication:
   - haloperidol, olanzapine or risperidone (*this patient is already taking this*)

- (± lorazepam)
- if after three doses 45–60 minutes apart there is no resolution, go to Step 3.
3. Consider IM treatment:
   - haloperidol (± lorazepam)
   - repeat up to three times at 30-minute intervals if needed.
4. Consider IV treatment:
   - site an IV cannula – ensure you have IV access
   - diazepam 10 mg over at least 5 minutes
   - repeat after 10 minutes if there is little or no effect (maximum three times)
5. Seek senior advice if there has been an inadequate response.

IMPORTANT NOTES

Have flumazenil to hand before administering benzodiazepines for rapid reversal of central sedative effects.

Monitor temperature, pulse, oxygen saturations, blood pressure and respiratory rate with IM/IV administration.
Give procyclidine (or similar) should acute dystonia (or other EPSE) develop.
Sometimes, going straight to parenteral administration to minimise risk to the patient and staff is necessary, but this needs to be a team decision. The use of IV antipsychotics is now not recommended. Discussion with a senior colleague or local expert would be advisable before considering this approach.

ASK WHETHER HE HAS ANY OTHER QUESTIONS

THANK HIM

FOR EXTRA MARKS

Transfer to a psychiatric ICU or a ward with a seclusion facility should be considered.

It is important to talk to the patient and explain what you are doing and why, as RT is enforced treatment that is often considered a violation by individuals. Following resolution, it is also important that the staff explain to the patient what happened and why various measures were taken.

COMPLICATIONS OF RT (*Clin Neuropharmacol* 1989; **4**: 233–48)

Local bruising, pain, extravasation
Respiratory complications
Cardiovascular complications
Hypotension
Seizures
NMS
Sudden death
EPSE

FURTHER READING

Hillard JR. Emergency treatment of acute psychosis. *J Clin Psychiatry* 1998; 59 (Suppl 1): 57–60, 61.

Taylor D, Paton C, Kerwin R. *The South London and Maudsley NHS Trust 2003 Prescribing Guidelines*, 7th edn. London: Martin Dunitz, 2003.

STATION 10: SEASONAL AFFECTIVE DISORDER

THE EXAMINER'S MARK SHEET	
Communication	SAD features
Empathy	Answering other questions
Mood assessment	Global rating

INTRODUCE YOURSELF

'Hello, nice to meet you. My name is Dr Smith.'

SET THE SCENE

'Thank you for coming today.'
'Could you tell me a little more about your mood and how you've been feeling recently?'

ASK FOR PERMISSION

'Would that be OK?'

TAKE A HISTORY OF SAD: KEY AREAS

Take a regular history for an affective disorder, eliciting the patient's symptoms. Establish a regular temporal relationship between autumn/winter and onset of symptoms. Does her mood lift as the days stretch out in spring/summer? Ask whether she has ever been away in Equatorial (hot) countries during the winter months and noticed that she did not feel depressed there.

Low mood can be of varying severity. Enquire about suicide ideation.
Fatiguability should be present.
Hyperphagia and *hypersomnia* are also noticeable.
Weight gain.

You should explain that many patients experience a seasonal pattern to their depressive illness. Some people call this SAD and believe it is a distinct entity because of its reversed biological features in winter. People with winter depression or SAD can remain in remission with holidays to the sun and light therapy. Treatment includes light therapy and conventional antidepressant treatments. Light therapy has been shown to be more effective in the morning rather than in the evening. It needs to be taken regularly (daily for 1–2 hours). Some people with SAD benefit from light boxes on their desks at work: 10 000-lux light is needed for any benefit. Light treatment should be started in early autumn or late summer.

SAD sufferers are thought to have circadian phase delay. The light therapy is thought to effect a phase advance, which alleviates the unwanted symptoms. Dawn-simulating light clocks are thought to help symptoms.
Travelling abroad to sunny climates in winter is the ultimate treatment.

ASK WHETHER SHE HAS ANY QUESTIONS

THANK HER

FOR EXTRA MARKS

Be aware that SAD is a controversial diagnosis thought by some to be a temporal coincidence between regular depression and the time of year. Cynics suggest that it is a creation of psychiatrists and the media. On balance, there is a continuum of symptoms in winter months, of which some individuals suffer much more than others.
Enquire about manic or hypomanic features during the summer months.
SAD is subsumed under recurrent depressive disorder in ICD-10 (F33).
Light boxes can be rented or purchased.

SUPPORT GROUPS

SAD Association: www.sada.org.uk

FURTHER READING

Eagles JM. Seasonal affective disorder. *Br J Psych* 2003; 182: 174–6.

STATION 11: TEMPORAL LOBE ASSESSMENT

THE EXAMINER'S MARK SHEET	
Communication/rapport	Bilateral testing
Dominant lobe	Answering any questions
Non-dominant lobe	Global rating

INTRODUCE YOURSELF

'Hello, nice to meet you. My name is Dr Smith.'

SET THE SCENE

Explain what your role is and ask whether she has noticed any problems, e.g. with her memory.

ASK FOR PERMISSION

Ask whether it would be OK if you went through some questions and tests that you ask everyone you see.

'Some of the things I'll be asking will be quite difficult, while others will be easier, but try not to worry if you make some mistakes.'

'Let me know if you are uncomfortable at any point or getting too tired.'

CLINICAL PROCEDURE: TEST THE FOLLOWING

Dominant lobe

Receptive dysphasia: obvious from conversation.

Alexia: ask her to read something.

Agraphia: ask her to write something.

Impaired learning and retention of verbal material: ask her to repeat an address – '42 West Register Street' – and to recall it after 5 minutes.

Non-dominant lobe

Visuospatial difficulties.

Anomia: ask her to name a wristwatch, strap and buckle.

Prosopagnosia: ask whether she recognises Queen Elizabeth on a £5 note.

Hemisomatopagnosia: belief that a limb is absent when it is not.

Impaired learning and retention of non-verbal material such as music or drawings: ask her to copy a drawing and to repeat from memory 5 minutes later:

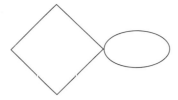

Bilateral lesions

Amnesic syndromes (Korsakoff's amnesia, Klüver–Bucy syndrome): assess short- and long-term memories.

THANK HER

FOR EXTRA MARKS

Consequences of neurological damage to temporal lobe structures: changes in behaviour/personality.
Enquire about change in the person: increased aggression, agitation or instability (limbic system).
Assess visual fields: contralateral homonymous upper quadrantanopia.
Other: depersonalisation
disturbance of sexual function
epileptic phenomena
psychotic disturbances akin to schizophrenia.

STATION 12: SSRIs: SEXUAL DYSFUNCTION

THE EXAMINER'S MARK SHEET	
Communication	Explanation/advice to couple
Empathy	Answering other questions
History of dysfunction	Global rating

INTRODUCE YOURSELF

'Hello my name's Dr Smith, I'm one of the psychiatrists.'

SET THE SCENE

'Could you tell me what is worrying you?'

'You seem very upset. What has happened?'

'I'm sorry to hear that that the medication has affected your sex life. Could you tell me what has changed?'

Be sure to have her husband's consent before discussing his case.

FIND OUT WHAT SHE ALREADY KNOWS

Were the couple counselled in the past about the potential medication side effects, particularly sexual side effects?

If not, then apologise and state that this should have happened. If the man has been on other antidepressants in the past, has he ever experienced other side effects?

She may be angry. Allow her to vent her frustration. Be supportive and empathetic. You are not failing the station if she 'loses her rag'. Keep calm and offer good advice.

INFORMATION ON SSRIS: SEXUAL DYSFUNCTION

Questions about one's sex life are personal and can be embarrassing for some people, so it is important to pose these questions in a sensitive and caring manner. Sexual side effects are common and serious, with the potential to cause damage to relationships.

An important question is whether any sexual side effects were present before the medication was taken. Sexual dysfunction can be a result of depression itself or entirely in relation to the treatment.

Ask about other side effects

Ask when the antidepressant was started and when the side effects began.

Ask whether anything has been done to date about the side effects.

Talk to her about the common side effects (nausea 25–35 per cent, vomiting, dyspepsia, insomnia, sexual dysfunction) of SSRIs.

Try to establish whether her husband is concerned about it. You will want to talk to him and decide together a course of action. It might transpire that he is less concerned than his wife. *He is the patient,* after all.

PLAN

The medication can be stopped, the dose lowered or another medication started. A discussion about risks versus benefits may follow.

Which medication the patient has been taking is important, as some antidepressant drugs are less likely to cause sexual dysfunction.

Cognitive and behavioural techniques can also be used to overcome sexual dysfunction, which is normally the remit of the sexual therapist.

ASK WHETHER SHE HAS ANY OTHER QUESTIONS

THANK HER

FOR EXTRA MARKS

Need to exclude medical causes (vascular, neurogenic, endocrine).
Medications that have been used for antidepressant-induced sexual dysfunction with varying success include:
- α2-adrenergic receptor antagonists, e.g. yohimbine
- serotonin 5HT2 or 5HT3 receptor antagonists, e.g. cyproheptadine, granisetron
- dopaminergic agents, e.g. amantadine, pramipexole.

The phosphodiesterase type-5 inhibitor sildenafil (Viagra®) is now used for erectile dysfunction in such cases.

FURTHER READING

Salerian AJ, Deibler WE, Vittone BJ, *et al.* Sildenafil for psychotropic-induced sexual dysfunction in 31 women and 61 men. *J Sex Marital Ther* 2000; **26:** 133–40.

EXAM 7

STATION 1

You are the psychiatrist on call. The medical SHO on call has come over to see you as she is concerned about an undernourished 18-year-old woman on a general medical ward. She thinks she may have anorexia nervosa, is concerned about her physical wellbeing, and is seeking your advice as she has very little knowledge in this area.

She wants to know:

How one makes a diagnosis of anorexia nervosa.
Whether there are any cardiovascular complications.
What the ECG is likely to show.

[advice on page 202]

STATION 2

A GP has referred this patient to you. She gave birth to a baby boy 2 months ago and over the past 5 weeks has been tearful and feeling 'low'. Her partner works in a very busy city job and comes back late in the evenings. She has no other children and no siblings. Her parents live in Spain and she sees them perhaps once a year. Several of her close friends have children and live in the area, but she has preferred not to socialise with them for several weeks now.

Elicit a psychiatric history from this woman.

[advice on page 205]

STATION 3

Perform an ECG on this patient.

[advice on page 208]

STATION 4

A 34-year-old heroin user has been injecting heroin for the past 6 months.

Assess the risks posed to his health by injecting.

[advice on page 210]

STATION 5

This patient who suffers from a bipolar disorder is currently manic.

Examine their manic behaviour.

[advice on page 213]

STATION 6

Take a history from this woman with social phobia, who is getting married in 3 weeks and complains of a worsening of her symptoms.

Explore the possible aetiological factors.

[advice on page 216]

STATION 7

Examine this patient's retinas.

[advice on page 218]

STATION 8

You receive a letter from a GP showing results suggestive of hypothyroidism in a patient who is taking lithium.

Explain these results to the patient, enquire about any symptoms, and perform a relevant examination.

[advice on page 220]

STATION 9

This 80-year-old woman has been brought to hospital by the police after she was found wandering the streets in the early hours of the morning. She appeared muddled but had not been drinking alcohol. She now says she is fine to go home. There is no additional information at the moment, other than knowing that she lives alone. The A&E doctor has already seen her and has cleared her medically. He thinks she may have dementia.

Assess whether this patient is safe to go home.

[advice on page 222]

STATION 10

A 28-year-old man with a diagnosis of a moderate depressive episode has been taking an antidepressant for 4 months. He has been feeling much better for the past 2 months and wants to stop his medication.

Speak to this man regarding his wish to stop medication, and advise him accordingly.

[advice on page 225]

STATION 11

Your consultant has asked you to assess this patient's personality.

[advice on page 228]

STATION 12

You are asked by the nursing staff to review this 43-year-old gentleman who has been exhibiting withdrawn behaviour.

[advice on page 230]

STATION 1: ANOREXIA NERVOSA

THE EXAMINER'S MARK SHEET	
Communication	ECG findings
Diagnostic criteria	Answering other questions
Cardiovascular complications	Global rating

INTRODUCE YOURSELF

'Hello, I'm Dr Smith. Nice to meet you.'
Stations dealing with colleagues do demand a more scientific approach and may feel like a viva. However, it is still an OSCE and you will gain marks for how you 'play the part' and deal with a professional.

SET THE SCENE

'Thanks for coming over. How is your patient?'
'Is she medically stable?'
'Can I ask how long she's been on the medical ward?'
'Why do you think she might have anorexia nervosa?'

FIND OUT WHAT SHE ALREADY KNOWS

'Have you ever seen anyone with an eating disorder before?'
Avoid embarrassing a colleague if they cannot remember their psychiatry.

INFORMATION ON ANOREXIA NERVOSA

Diagnosis

Explain that a diagnosis of AN is based upon the ICD-10 diagnostic criteria. For a definite diagnosis, the following are required:

Body weight 15 per cent below that expected, or a BMI of 17.5 or less.
Self-induced weight loss by avoiding 'fattening foods'. One or more of the following may also be present: self-induced vomiting, purging, excessive exercise, use of appetite suppressants and/or diuretics.
Body image distortion.
Widespread endocrine disorder involving the hypothalamic-pituitary-gonadal axis (amenorrhoea in women, reduced libido and potency in men).
If prepubertal, then the sequence of prepubertal events is delayed or even arrested.

Cardiovascular complications

Bradycardia (commonest):   < 60 beats per minute in 80 per cent of patients
Tachycardia
Hypotension: < 90/60 mm Hg, often due to chronic volume
                                           depletion
Ventricular arrhythmias: electrolyte disturbances from diuretic/laxative abuse
Cardiac failure: may be a terminal event

ECG

A variety of ECG changes, including sinus bradycardia, ST depression and a prolonged QT interval. Regular ECG monitoring is recommended, especially if severely undernourished.

OTHER POSSIBLE QUESTIONS

What about gastrointestinal problems?

Enamel and dentine erosion if vomiting frequently
Benign enlargement of the parotid gland
Oesophagitis, erosions, ulcers
Oesophageal rupture
Gastric dilation after refeeding (care!)
Delayed gastric emptying
Constipation: inadequate food intake and fluid depletion from diuretics/laxatives
Diarrhoea: due to stimulating laxatives

Is neutropenia common?

A pancytopenia is common in severe AN
Leucopenia in up to two-thirds of patients
Mild anaemia and thrombocytopenia can occur in up to one-third of patients
Repeat FBC and exclude organic causes

Is urinalysis important?

It can be helpful. Proteinuria can be detected. If severe or chronic, the renal physicians should be involved.

ASK WHETHER SHE HAS ANY OTHER QUESTIONS

THANK HER

FOR EXTRA MARKS

BMI = <u>(weight in kilograms)</u>

      (height in metres)^2.

Benign enlargement of the parotid gland (25 per cent of cases of bulimia).
Oesophageal rupture (Boerhaave's syndrome) is a complication associated
with vomiting after meals, i.e. after bingeing.

*For formal specialist advice, recommend seeking the opinion of an eating
disorders specialist service.*

There may be morphological changes in red blood cells – ancanthocytes (spur
cells).

FURTHER READING

Klein DA, Walsh BT. Eating disorders: clinical features and pathophysiology.
Physiol Behav 2004; **81**: 359–74.

STATION 2: PERINATAL DISORDER

THE EXAMINER'S MARK SHEET	
Communication	Relevant mental state
Empathy	Answering other questions
Relevant history	Global rating

INTRODUCE YOURSELF

'Hello, I'm Dr Smith. Nice to meet you.'

SET THE SCENE

Ask an open question about how she has been feeling recently.

A supportive statement will demonstrate your understanding of her situation and encourage good rapport: 'The weeks after delivery are often extremely stressful.' 'It's very common to feel this way after the baby is born.'

ASK FOR PERMISSION

'Could we talk a little more about this?'

Then home in by using more closed questions where appropriate.

TAKE A HISTORY OF PERINATAL DISORDER: KEY AREAS

Of note, the ICD-10 does not classify puerperal disorders separately unless they do not meet the criteria for disorders classified elsewhere. Section F53, *mental and behavioural disorders associated with the puerperium, not elsewhere classified*, can be used in such circumstances.

This station is testing your knowledge of the common mental disorders associated with the puerperium. You cannot take a comprehensive psychiatric history in 6 minutes. You should plan to cover the likely differential diagnoses:

Postnatal blues
Postnatal depression
Puerperal psychosis

Postnatal blues

Enquire about tearfulness, low mood, emotional lability and confusion.

Ask about onset – usually a few days after delivery.

Usually resolves within a few days.

Up to half of all mothers are affected.

Management comprises support and reassurance. Little or no support from the partner or family, as in this case, may play a major role in poor adjustment to new life circumstances.

Postnatal depression

Onset usually within 3 months of delivery.
10 to 15 per cent of mothers are affected.
Likely to be similar to non-puerperal depressive episode.
Enquire about low mood, reduced interests, low self-esteem, tearfulness, anxiety, concerns about the baby and its health, coping with the new routine, whether she is breastfeeding and if so whether it has been problematic.
Ask about *suicidal ideation* or *wish to harm others, especially the baby.*
Ask about previous psychiatric history of depression.

Has the midwife or doctor asked her to complete a questionnaire that asked about her mood (Edinburgh Postnatal Depression Scale)? This ten-item questionnaire would be worth completing at some point, but you would not need to memorise this.
Management options:

Counselling, self-help groups, psychotherapy
Antidepressants (*seek advice*)
Admission (to mother and baby unit if bed available)

ECT is not contraindicated, but should be considered only if other options have failed or the mother is extremely unwell.

Puerperal psychosis

0.2 per cent of live births
Increased risk especially during the first 2 weeks after delivery
Usually abrupt onset
Ask about mood, hallucinations and delusions
Fluctuation in mental state, with perplexity, restlessness, anxiety
Enquire about manic features (affective psychosis most common), including severe insomnia in the absence of the baby crying
Ask about previous psychiatric history

Management options:

Admission is often necessary in the interests of safety
Mother and baby unit would be best
Medication: lithium, if manic component (breastfeeding to be stopped)
                neuroleptic, after discussion with specialist unit and drug
                information
                antidepressants
Supportive counselling/psychotherapy
ECT

Risk

Always consider the risk to the mother and the baby.
Any medication prescribed needs to be considered carefully if the mother is breastfeeding.
The woman's partner needs education and support.

ASK WHETHER SHE HAS ANY QUESTIONS

THANK HER

FOR EXTRA MARKS

Other possible related OSCEs:

Assess this woman, who is tearful having had a baby several weeks ago
Puerperal psychosis
Lithium and pregnancy
Medications and breastfeeding

Five to ten per cent of women attending obstetric clinics have psychiatric disturbance (*Br J Psychiatry* 1984; 144: 35–47).
Women with a history of BPAD have up to a 25 per cent chance of having an affective psychosis following childbirth.

FURTHER READING

Seyfried LS, Marcus SM. Postpartum mood disorders. *Int Rev Psychiatry* 2003; 15: 231–42.

STATION 3: PERFORM AN ECG

THE EXAMINER'S MARK SHEET	
Communication	Acquiring the ECG
Patient consideration	Answering other questions
Electrode application	Global rating

INTRODUCE YOURSELF

'Hello, I'm Dr Smith. Nice to meet you.'

EXPLAIN WHAT YOU HAVE BEEN ASKED TO DO

Explain to the patient (probably a mannequin) that you would like to take a tracing of their heart.

ASK FOR PERMISSION

'Would that be OK?'

'Let me know if you are uncomfortable at any point.'

Explain that there is no pain involved and describe briefly what you will be doing.

CLINICAL PROCEDURE

Equipment

Make sure that you have all the necessary equipment:

Four limb leads
Six chest leads
Electrode stickers
ECG machine and mains supply

Procedure

Attach the electrode stickers. If the patient is an actor rather than a mannequin, try to avoid bony points and hairy areas. Know the anatomical landmarks for chest leads V1–V6 and where to apply limb leads. Know how to count down to the fourth intercostal space from the manubrio-sternal junction.

Limb leads should be labelled or colour-coded:

Right arm: red
Left arm: yellow
Right leg: black
Left leg: green

Chest leads:

V1: fourth intercostal space, right of sternum
V2: fourth intercostal space, left of sternum
V3: mid-way between V2 and V4
V4: left fifth intercostal space, mid-clavicular line
V5: anterior axillary line, level with V4
V6: mid-axillary line, level with V4

Ask the patient to relax and lie still while you acquire the ECG tracing. Wait for about 10 seconds while the patient relaxes before recording the trace.

THANK THE PATIENT

FOR EXTRA MARKS

The patient should be relaxed, warm and free from any muscular effort.
Consider using a chaperone with a female patient.
If the patient has a tremor of a hand or limb, the limb lead can be sited further up to assist the trace.
Always label the ECG with name, date, etc.
Remove the electrode stickers from the patient.
Interpret the ECG if you have time, and report back the findings to the patient.

STATION 4: HAZARDS OF INJECTING ILLICIT DRUGS

THE EXAMINER'S MARK SHEET	
Communication	Harm minimisation (advice)
Empathy	Answering other questions
Injecting risks	Global rating

INTRODUCE YOURSELF

'Hello, I'm Dr Smith. Nice to meet you.'

SET THE SCENE

'I wanted to talk to you about heroin and what the effects have been on your life.'

FIND OUT WHAT THEY ALREADY KNOW

'Are you aware of the dangers associated with using heroin?'
'Have you ever run into problems using drugs?'

INFORMATION ON INJECTING HAZARDS

This is an unlikely station, but it is useful for the sake of complete preparation, as the issues can come up as part of another OSCE.

Ask where he injects

The site of injection is very important, as some areas are extremely dangerous. Injecting in the groin and neck is more dangerous due to the presence of large nerves and arteries. In chronic opiate injectors, injecting in these body areas is common.

Assess his knowledge of injecting hazards

Most chronic addicts will know the arrangement of anatomical structures in the groin. However, not all do – if they are likely to continue injecting, then it is an opportunity to inform the patient. The vein is most medial.

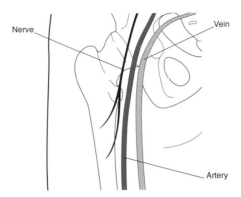

NAVY: nerve, artery, vein, Y-fronts.

This mnemonic allows one to remember that the vein is most medial, nearest to the underwear (Y-fronts).

Risks of injecting:

Infection (bacterial, HIV, hepatitis)
Overdose
Vein damage
Blood clots
Increased level of dependence compared with other routes of administration

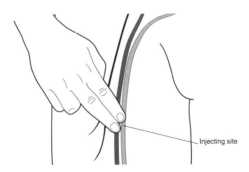

Give correct injecting technique instructions: although controversial, harm-minimisation initiatives play an important role in the addiction field. If an addict has physical evidence of injecting and refuses to stop, then imparting knowledge might reduce harm related to this activity.

'Find the pulse in the groin, put your middle finger there and keep it there.'
'Put your index finger tightly alongside your middle finger and choose an injecting site towards the centre of your body immediately next to your index finger.'

This should ensure that he misses the femoral nerve or artery.

Give information on artery damage

One can expect severe pain if an artery is hit.
The plunger of the syringe is pushed back.
Do not continue to inject.
Lie down and apply firm pressure.
Call an ambulance and get help.

ASK WHETHER HE HAS ANY QUESTIONS

THANK HIM

FOR EXTRA MARKS

When blood supply to the leg is blocked, *gangrene* occurs.
Keep injection sites healthy.
Give veins a chance to recover.
Beware of swapping between groins: infection may spread.
Wash hands well before injecting.

HELP/ADVICE

Needle exchanges (don't share needles!)
Leaflets from dependency units on injecting and hazards

FURTHER READING

Wodak A. Managing illicit drug use: a practical guide. *Drugs* 1994; **47**: 446–57.

STATION 5: MANIC PATIENT

THE EXAMINER'S MARK SHEET

Communication	Risk issues
Relevant history	Answering other questions
Mental state	Global rating

INTRODUCE YOURSELF

'Hello, I'm Dr Smith. Nice to meet you.'

SET THE SCENE

Begin with a general opening:
'I wanted to talk to you about how you've been feeling in yourself recently.'

ASK FOR PERMISSION

'Would that be OK?'
'Has anything been worrying you?'

ASSESSMENT OF MANIA: KEY AREAS

In reality, it is difficult to interview a floridly manic patient and gather reliable information. In the exam situation, it is likely that the actor will try to appear distractible and overactive, with flight of ideas, punning or clanging.
It will soon become apparent how manic the actor is likely to be and this will dictate which course to take. Try not to become stressed if you are unable to cover all the areas that you would hope to.

History of events

Significant events leading up to the current episode should be explored (any precipitants?).
If the patient is exhibiting flight of ideas, then it will be hard to keep them on one topic. It is important to try to keep control of the interview without irritating the patient.

Relevant mental state

'I wanted to ask you about your mood of late.'
'Do you think you have been cheerful recently?'
'Have you been excessively cheerful?'

Then attempt to elicit as many of the features of mania as possible:

'Have you felt full of energy or full of exciting ideas?'
'How has your sleep been?'

'Sometimes, when people become very cheerful in mood, they can overspend. Have you been spending much of late? Any luxury purchases? More than you can afford?'
'Have you felt more irritable lately?'
'Have you had more arguments than usual?'
'Have you been using more alcohol and drugs than usual?'
'Do you feel you've been disinhibited with other people?'
'Have you had any recent short-term relationships or sexual relationships that you feel are out of character for you?'
(These questions must be posed in a tactful manner).

'Have you been attending work in the past days and weeks?'
'Have you felt super-efficient at work or at home?'
'Have you felt as though you had special powers or amazing talents?'

Enquire about abnormal perceptions (psychosis) and delusional beliefs.

Medication
It is important to get an idea of the medication, if any, that the patient has been taking and whether there has been discontinuation of treatment, which is a frequent cause of relapse:
'Do you take any regular medication?'

Risk assessment
It is important to consider the patient's risk-taking behaviour (some issues will have come to light from the MSE).

ASK WHETHER THEY HAVE ANY QUESTIONS

THANK THEM

FOR EXTRA MARKS

You should be able to determine from the above whether the patient is manic or hypomanic (ICD-10).

When assessing a manic patient, you should also enquire about depressive symptomatology (mixed-state/cycling BPAD?):

'Sometimes, when people feel cheerful for extended periods of time, there can be periods in between where the mood becomes very low.'
'Have you experienced any low mood recently?'
'You say you have been feeling low in yourself. Sometimes, when the mood becomes increasingly low, people feel like harming themselves. Have you had thoughts of harming yourself?'
'Sometimes, when mood becomes very low, people have thoughts of dying. This can be very distressing. Have you had thoughts of wanting to die?'
'Have you made any plans of harming yourself?'
'Have you told anyone of these plans?'

FURTHER READING

Hirschfeld RM, Vornik LA. Recognition and diagnosis of bipolar disorder. *J Clin Psychiatry* 2004; **65** (Suppl 15): 5–9.

STATION 6: SOCIAL PHOBIA

THE EXAMINER'S MARK SHEET	
Communication	Aetiological factors
Empathy	Answering other questions
Social phobia: history	Global rating

INTRODUCE YOURSELF

'Hello, I'm Dr Smith. Nice to meet you.'

SET THE SCENE

'I understand you're getting married in a few weeks. Congratulations!'
'Can I ask how you feel about the wedding?'

ASK FOR PERMISSION

'Would that be OK?'

TAKE A HISTORY OF SOCIAL PHOBIA: KEY AREAS

Display an empathetic disposition.

Confirm the diagnosis

Social phobia is an umbrella term for a number of similar conditions based on shyness and a lack of confidence. The picture, however, can range from a phobic reaction of interacting in small groups to eating in public. In which situations does she get anxious and what does she tend to avoid? Explore the psychological, behavioural and autonomic symptoms.
A diagnosis demands the following (ICD-10 guidelines):

Symptoms must be a primary manifestation of anxiety and not secondary to other symptoms, such as delusions or obsessional thoughts.
Anxiety is restricted or predominates in social situations.
The phobic situation is avoided.

Assess the severity of the disorder

Examine the impact of the anxiety on her daily life.
What, if anything, does she fear about her wedding? It is likely that there is some anxiety concerning:

Being observed by others (centre of attention)
Eating at the wedding
Having to speak in public
Having to interact with the guests

Is there anticipatory anxiety?
Is there a comorbid diagnosis (depression)?

Aetiology

Primary: no other psychiatric condition present
Secondary: nearly always secondary to depression

Ask about the onset of the condition: it may have been preceded by a humiliating event.
It is important to differentiate between normal shyness and avoidant personality traits. People can display shyness and not have social phobia or be personality-disordered.
Does she use any substances to relieve anxiety, e.g. alcohol, benzodiazepines or illicit drugs?
The phobia may have been present for some time in another form.

ASK WHETHER SHE HAS ANY QUESTIONS

THANK HER

FOR EXTRA MARKS

Men : women 1 : 1.
Social phobias often start in adolescence.
Often associated with agoraphobia and depression.
Be aware of the difference between social phobia and social anxiety. We all get anxious in varying amounts, most of which is within normal boundaries. The anxiety should be severe for a diagnosis of social phobia.

FURTHER READING

Kennerley H. *Managing Anxiety: A Training Manual*. Oxford: Oxford University Press, 1990.

STATION 7: FUNDOSCOPY

THE EXAMINER'S MARK SHEET	
Communication	Presentation of findings
Patient consideration	Answering other questions
Technique	Global rating

INTRODUCE YOURSELF

'Hello, I'm Dr Smith. Nice to meet you.'

EXPLAIN WHAT YOU HAVE BEEN ASKED TO DO

Explain that you would like to examine their eyes and that this involves a bright light.
'If it is uncomfortable at any point, let me know.'

ASK FOR PERMISSION

'Would that be OK?'

CLINICAL PROCEDURE

Remember to treat a mannequin as if it were a patient.

Set the ophthalmoscope lens to zero.
Check that it works.
Tell the patient to fixate on a distant target.
Start at arm's length and shine the white light at each eye in turn to elicit the red reflex. Its absence should alert you to the possibility of an opacity (cataract) between the two chambers.
Examine the patient's right eye with your right eye and then their left eye with your left eye. This enables the patient to remain fixated on the distant object.
Ask the patient to look straight at the light to enable you to examine the macula.

Optic disc

Locate and bring into focus.
Look for size, blurred disc edge, cupping (glaucoma), new vessels (diabetic retinopathy), pale disc (e.g. optic atrophy).

Blood vessels

Arteries are narrower and brighter and have a reflective pale streak.
Start at the disc and follow the vessels out to look for hypertensive changes (A-V nipping) and atherosclerotic changes.

Fundus

Look for haemorrhages, exudates, cotton-wool spots, new vessel formation, and micro-aneurysms.

Be familiar with:

Papilloedema: blurred disc edge, haemorrhages, hard exudates (late feature), cotton-wool spots (due to retinal infarction).

Diabetic retinopathy: micro-aneurysms, small haemorrhages, exudates, cotton-wool spots, new vessel formation (proliferative diabetic retinopathy).

Hypertensive retinopathy: silver wiring, A-V nipping, haemorrhages, cotton-wool spots, disc swelling if malignant.

Glaucoma: optic disc enlargement, undermining of the disc margins, blood vessel bowing (advanced).

Comment on the main features as you examine them, or complete your examination and then turn to the examiner to present your findings.

THANK THE PATIENT

FOR EXTRA MARKS

If asked to 'examine the eyes', remember to perform full examination of the second cranial (optic) nerve, as in the CNS exam.

Describe any features with reference to a clock face and optic disc size: 'There are soft exudates at three o'clock, two disc diameters away from the disc.'

Explain that, ideally, you would like to examine the retinas in a dark room or dilate the pupils to get a better view (one per cent cyclopentolate).

Learn the appearance of the common eye pathologies.

Be familiar with retinal artery and vein occlusion, macular degeneration, optic atrophy and MS.

STATION 8: LITHIUM AND HYPOTHYROIDISM

THE EXAMINER'S MARK SHEET	
Communication	Thyroid examination
Explanation	Answering other questions
Symptoms	Global rating

INTRODUCE YOURSELF
'Hello, I'm Dr Smith. Nice to meet you.'

SET THE SCENE
'We've had the results of the thyroid tests you had recently.'

FIND OUT WHAT THEY ALREADY KNOW
'Did your GP talk to you about the results?'

INFORMATION ON LITHIUM AND THYROID DYSFUNCTION

Explanation
'The results show that the thyroid is a bit underactive.'

'This is why we monitor thyroid function regularly, as there is a risk that lithium can interfere with the thyroid gland.'

'It's nothing to be too worried about, but it is something we will need to monitor and correct.'

'The thyroid gland produces hormones necessary for bodily function, in particular metabolism. In hypothyroidism, the hormone levels are low due to underproduction of the hormones by the gland. This occurs in about five per cent of people taking lithium. The condition normally comes on slowly, so you may not have noticed any symptoms. I have noticed from your blood results that your levels of thyroid hormones are low. The good news is that the condition can be treated effectively by replacing the hormone in the form of a tablet called thyroxine.'

Clinical symptoms
'May I ask you whether you have experienced a lack of energy?'

Enquire also about cold intolerance, slowness in thought and action, hoarseness, weight gain, changes in hair and skin texture, pins and needles and constipation. Ask about mood, in particular depression.

Thyroid examination

Refer to Exam 2, Station 4 for full examination.

Inspect the neck, looking at the thyroid gland.
A thyroid examination should be performed standing behind the patient.
It can be difficult to see the thyroid gland in a healthy person.
An enlarged thyroid gland will definitely be visible (goitre).
Identify the cricoid cartilage with the fingers of both hands.
Move downwards two or three tracheal rings while *palpating* for the isthmus.
Move laterally from the mid-line, while palpating for the lobes of the thyroid.
Note the size, symmetry and position of the lobes, as well as the presence of any nodules.
Percussion.
Auscultation.

ASK THE PATIENT WHETHER THEY HAVE ANY QUESTIONS

THANK THE PATIENT

FOR EXTRA MARKS

Five per cent of patients taking lithium for 18 months or more will develop hypothyroidism. Females are more at risk than males.

Investigations performed to substantiate thyroid disease include:

Ultrasound of neck and thyroid
Blood tests; thyroid function
Radioactive thyroid scan
Fine-needle aspiration biopsy
Chest X-ray
CT or MRI scan

FURTHER READING

Kleiner J, Altshuler L, Hendrick V, Hershman JM. Lithium-induced subclinical hypothyroidism: review of the literature and guidelines for treatment. *J Clin Psychiatry* 1999; **60**: 249–55.

STATION 9: DEMENTIA: WANDERING

THE EXAMINER'S MARK SHEET	
Communication	Cognitive assessment
Empathy	Answering other questions
Risk	Global rating

INTRODUCE YOURSELF

'Hello, I'm Dr Smith. Nice to meet you.'
Explain that you are one of the psychiatrists and that you have been asked to see her.

SET THE SCENE

'I wanted to talk to you about what happened this morning.'

ASK FOR PERMISSION

'Would that be OK?'

ASSESS WHETHER THE PATIENT CAN RETURN HOME: KEY AREAS

Two main issues:

Risk
Possible dementia diagnosis

To tackle both fully in the time available is challenging, so the advice is to always stick to the question asked.

First, find out about the risks involved.
If time allows, perform a full or abbreviated cognitive assessment.
If the patient is too cognitively impaired to give meaningful responses, then move swiftly to the MMSE.

Risk

Ask what happened this morning – can she remember any details?
Does she appear appropriately concerned about what happened? (It can be extremely distressing to lose one's memory, even temporarily.)
If not, then explain your concerns about the risks she faced. Does she seem to understand? (Insight?)
Does she remember her home address?
Does she live alone? (You would want to speak to anyone living at home with her, her neighbours or a warden if she lives in supported accommodation – how has she been managing there?)

Does she have any next of kin or friends whom you would be able to talk to?
Are there any healthcare (or allied) professionals (CMHT for older adults, CPN,
social worker, occupational therapist, day centre) involved?
Has anything like this happened before? (You would want to corroborate this
with A&E, the police and her family doctor.)
It is important to find out about her living conditions (food, hygiene,
gas/electricity). Is she looking after herself appropriately?
It is important to note her current level of personal care
(?kempt/undernourished).

Also:

Is she psychotic? (Presence of abnormal perceptions or delusions –
paranoid/persecutory/command?)
History of alcohol or substance misuse?
History of falling over?
History of harming herself or others?
History of behavioural disturbances (in public or at home)?

Is she prescribed any regular medication, e.g. acetylcholinesterase inhibitors,
antipsychotics, antidepressants? Is she taking them appropriately?

Cognitive assessment

Cognitive assessment (MMSE or similar), as described in Exam 3, Station 2.

Admitting the patient to hospital would depend upon the information gathered
during the interview. Even if she is cognitively impaired, the patient should be
part of the process and updated continually. Admitting an elderly person with
dementia can be extremely distressing for the patient, and so you must provide
her with appropriate reassurance.

ASK WHETHER SHE HAS ANY QUESTIONS

THANK HER

FOR EXTRA MARKS

Although she has been cleared medically and there would be no time in this OSCE, in reality you would still want to perform a full neurological assessment and examine her for evidence of a fall or head injury. It would be important to exclude an acute confusional state (delirium).

If a patient's level of risk necessitates admission, then you might need to consider using the 1983 Mental Health Act. Currently for patients who lack capacity to consent but do not dissent, the House of Lords' overturning of *R. v. Bournewood Community and Mental Health NHS Trust ex parte L. House of Lords judgment* (25 June 1998) allows admission without recourse to the Mental Health Act. This ruling may change again in the future.

Fluctuating attention in Lewy body dementia and vascular dementia can contribute to confusion.

FURTHER READING

Lai CK, Arthur DG. Wandering behaviour in people with dementia. *J Adv Nurs* 2003; 44: 173–82.

STATION 10: STOPPING MEDICATION

THE EXAMINER'S MARK SHEET	
Communication	Advice on stopping and other options
Risks/benefits	Answering other questions
Relevant mental state	Global rating

INTRODUCE YOURSELF

'Hello, I'm Dr Smith. Nice to meet you.'

SET THE SCENE

'You've been taking the antidepressant now for 4 months – is that right?'
'How have you been feeling in terms of your mood?'
Thank him for coming to talk to you about stopping the medication, rather than just stopping.

FIND OUT WHAT HE KNOWS ALREADY

'Do you know much about antidepressants and stopping treatment?'

INFORMATION ON STOPPING ANTIDEPRESSANTS

He needs to be made aware of the following:

Risks of stopping:
- relapse of mood disorder, with associated impact on relationships, employment, finances, social and family life, and more
- discontinuation symptoms if stopped abruptly.

Benefits of stopping:
- no inconvenience of pills to take
- avoid side effects.

Clarify the situation

Has this man really been feeling good for the past 2 months, or are there other reasons for wanting to stop the medication?

Increased depressive and suicidal symptoms can lead patients to want to give up medication.
Enquire about his mood and biological features.
Is this his first episode of depression? Some patients describe a pattern of relapsing mood when they discontinue treatment. These are candidates for longer-term/maintenance treatment.

Medication

Ask which medication he has been taking, at what dose, for how long and at what time of the day.

Get an idea of medication adherence. Has he taken the medication at all?

Ask about side effects. They can be uncomfortable and may lead patients to discontinue treatment.

Usual practice

Explain the *risk of relapse* and *discontinuation symptoms* when stopping abruptly. Medication is best tapered off slowly. This will depend on the medication itself, but is usually over 4 weeks.

It is generally recommended that in depression, medication is continued for at least 6 months and for up to 12 months following resolution of symptoms. Stopping prematurely may risk relapse. You need to explain this and also that treatment should be longer if this is recurrent depression.

Alternative medication

Explain that there are a number of different classes of antidepressants, which act in different ways and have different side-effect profiles. If he is still depressed, then it may be that a different medication will be tolerated better. Sometimes, it takes a while to find the right medication for an individual.

Psychotherapy

If it transpires that he remains depressed but refuses medication, you can discuss psychotherapeutic approaches. He may be more amenable to 'talking therapy'. Explain that there is good evidence to suggest that psychotherapy together with medication is the most effective antidepressant approach.

ASK WHETHER HE HAS ANY QUESTIONS

THANK HIM

FOR EXTRA MARKS

Fifty per cent of patients will experience a relapse if they stop their medication as soon as they feel better.

ECT is a very effective antidepressant that usually works quite quickly. It is more acceptable than medication to some people.

When enquiring about antidepressant side effects, don't forget sexual dysfunction. This is much more common than previously thought.

It can be quite useful in situations where the clinician feels that the patient is depressed but the patient disagrees for the patient to complete a Beck Depression Inventory (BDI) and for the clinician to complete a Hamilton Depression Rating Scale.

There is a lot of anxiety about antidepressants in the media currently. Many people would rather avoid taking these medications, and this is something the patient may want to discuss.

FURTHER READING

Geddes JR, Carney SM, Davies C, *et al.* Relapse prevention with antidepressant drug treatment in depressive disorders: a systematic review. *Lancet* 2003; **361**: 653–61.

STATION 11: PERSONALITY

THE EXAMINER'S MARK SHEET	
Communication	Traits elicited
Rapport	Answering other questions
Components of personality	Global rating

INTRODUCE YOURSELF
'Hello, I'm Dr Smith. Nice to meet you.'

SET THE SCENE
Explain that you would like to get an idea of what kind of person they are and how they might react in different situations.

ASK FOR PERMISSION
Ask whether it would be OK to ask some questions that you ask everyone you see.

ASSESS THIS PATIENT'S PERSONALITY: KEY AREAS
Try to get an overall impression and scan for personality traits.
Ask about the following:

Character
'Can you tell me what kind of person you are?'
'How would you describe your own personality?'
Reserved/timid
Shy/self-conscious/anxious (avoidant)
Fussy/difficult/meticulous/punctual (anankastic)
Selfish/self-centred
Centre of attention (histrionic)
Attitudes of others – 'How would people that know you describe your personality?'
Attitudes to others – 'What do you think of other people, for example your friends or people at work?'

Habits
Risk-taking behaviour (± criminal behaviour) (dissocial)
Smoking, alcohol, drugs

Reactions to stress
'How would you cope in an extremely stressful situation, for example if you lost your job or somebody was rude to you?'

Temperament

'What are you like if you get angry?'
'Has your temper ever got you into trouble?'(dissocial)
'Do you ever think you are irresponsible?' (dissocial)
'Do you get into lots of arguments?' (impulsive)
'How do you respond to criticism?' (anxious/paranoid)
'Are you ever very emotional?' (histrionic/borderline)

Friendships and relationships

'Have they been enduring?'
'Do you have many friends?' (schizoid)
'How do you get on with other people?' (paranoid)
'Do you trust other people?' (impulsive/paranoid)
'Have you ever had serious arguments with a partner?' 'How did you handle this?' (borderline)
'Do you think you depend on other people to get by?'(dependent)

Fantasy thinking

'What do you dream of or wish for?'
'Do you ever daydream about things? Tell me more about this.' (schizoid)

Prevailing mood

'What is your mood like for most of the time?' (predominantly cheery/gloomy)

ASK THE PATIENT WHETHER THEY HAVE ANY QUESTIONS

THANK THEM

FOR EXTRA MARKS

If you are asked whether the patient has a personality disorder, it would be prudent to say that it is difficult to make this diagnosis after one meeting and without the benefit of more collateral information. However, do mention if they have traits of a particular personality disorder (ICD-10).

Chart fame: Character
　　　　　　　*H*abits
　　　　　　　*R*eaction to stress
　　　　　　　*T*emperament
　　　　　　　*F*antasy thinking
　　　　　　　*M*ood (prevailing)
　　　　　　　*E*nduring relationships

STATION 12: WITHDRAWN BEHAVIOUR

THE EXAMINER'S MARK SHEET	
Communication	Eliciting psychopathology
Empathy	Answering other questions
Appropriate history	Global rating

INTRODUCE YOURSELF

'Hello, I'm Dr Smith. Nice to meet you.'

SET THE SCENE

'I wanted to find out how you've been feeling recently.'

'Has anything been worrying you?'

'The nursing staff have noticed that you seem to be withdrawn. Is there a reason for this?'

ASK FOR PERMISSION

'Would that be OK?'

WITHDRAWN BEHAVIOUR: KEY AREAS

This is a challenging station. There is a wide differential diagnosis for this type of presentation, and the actor is likely to be ungenerous with information. Use your knowledge of a general psychiatric assessment to briefly cover most bases. In other words, quite quickly you should be able to ask filter questions to establish whether this is depression, psychosis, chronic schizophrenia or cognitive impairment.

The possible causes of withdrawn behaviour will guide you. Therefore, when considering depression, you will ask about low mood, reduced energy, poor motivation, poor concentration, loss of enjoyment, etc.

DIFFERENTIAL DIAGNOSES

Depression/psychotic state, leading to withdrawal because of retardation (depression) or hallucinations (psychosis)

Residual/chronic schizophrenia

Dementia

Delirious state secondary to an infection (e.g. UTI)

CVA (stroke) – this can lead to aphasia, i.e. an inability to comprehend or express speech or written language

Intoxication due to prescribed or illicit drugs and alcohol

Learning disability may lead to withdrawn behaviour

Hearing impairment can lead to a reduction in observed communication

Personality disorder is a potential cause of withdrawn behaviour. Paranoid, anxious or schizoid features of personality may be contributing to withdrawn behaviour. However, on the basis of a quick interview during an OSCE, it is not possible to diagnose personality disorder. Speak instead about possible 'personality traits'.

Malingering, although not common, is a potential cause of withdrawn behaviour, particularly in prisoners.

Once you have a likely diagnosis, the interview can follow its natural course.

ASK WHETHER HE HAS ANY QUESTIONS

THANK HIM

FOR EXTRA MARKS

The first minute of this station is key. Approaching a withdrawn patient is a core skill in psychiatry. A modified introduction in which increased empathy is shown is what is required, paying attention to risk (e.g. patient lashing out).

An infective or neurological aetiology would require a *physical examination*.

EXAM 8

STATION 1

A nurse pages you, asking whether you could attend urgently to a patient who has collapsed on the ward. When you arrive, you are told he is unconscious and not breathing. There is no defibrillator available.

How will you proceed?

[advice on page 238]

STATION 2

This 22-year-old dancer has been re-admitted informally through her local psychiatric outpatients' department with a relapse of an eating disorder. She has a 3-year history of low weight. Her weight now is 29.5 kg and she is 1.62 m tall. She stopped menstruating 12 months ago. There has been one previous medical admission with gastritis and mild haematemesis and one psychiatric admission for 3 months last year. Her weight during that admission increased from 29 kg to 37 kg.

You are seeing her on the ward, where you have been asked by your consultant to find out about her dietary and weight history.

[advice on page 240]

STATION 3

This is an ECG tracing from a 45-year-old gentleman who has been taking neuroleptic medication for 7 years. He has been admitted to an inpatients' unit following a recent deterioration in his mental state. As part of a routine assessment, the nursing staff perform an ECG. They ask you whether the ECG tracing is normal.

Please report back on the findings of the ECG.

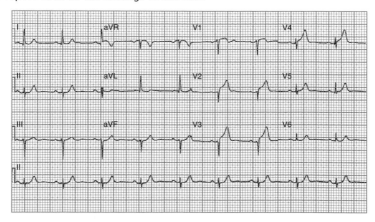

[advice on page 242]

STATION 4

This 26-year-old man is presenting reporting use of stimulants.

Take a history from him, ascertaining whether he is dependent.

[advice on page 245]

STATION 5

This 49-year-old gentleman with a long history of alcohol misuse is attending the community clinic. His appointment was not until next week, and several members of staff believe he has memory difficulties.

Assess this gentleman for Korsakoff's syndrome.

[advice on page 247]

STATION 6

This man has been prescribed an antidepressant by his family doctor. He wants to talk to you first before starting treatment.

Discuss the issues around commencing antidepressant medication.

[advice on page 249]

STATION 7

This 27-year-old woman is a patient of yours. She has a schizophrenic illness and has been treated over the past 5 years with several different neuroleptics. She has been on amisulpride for a year now, which she seems to get along with, as it has not made her drowsy or dizzy. She has asked to see you as she has something rather embarrassing to tell you. Over the past 2 weeks, she has noticed what she thinks is milk seeping from her breasts. She is worried about it and assures you she is not pregnant, as she has not had a boyfriend or slept with anyone for over a year.

Explain to the patient what you think is going on.

[advice on page 251]

STATION 8

A 25-year-old man is seen in the A&E department. He has self-harmed by taking an overdose the night before. He wishes to be discharged; he is insisting that he is well, that he was stupid and that it will not happen again. You notice ligature marks on his neck.

Assess the risk that this man poses to himself and others.

[advice on page 253]

STATION 9

You decide you wish to admit the patient from the previous OSCE station, as you have concerns about his safety.

Discuss with the consultant on the phone what it is you would like to do.

[advice on page 255]

STATION 10

This 19-year-old black African woman recently presented for the first time to psychiatric services. She had just started a media studies course at university when her personality seemed to change. She became increasingly inappropriate, paranoid about a fellow student and confused. After considerable deterioration, she was detained under the Mental Health Act and diagnosed with a psychotic illness. On the ward, she was agitated and aggressive. Physical examination, routine bloods and urinalysis on admission were all normal.

After 3 months on the ward, there has been no improvement despite treatment with olanzapine and then risperidone, both at therapeutic doses.
She is now disoriented for time and place. When seen in the doctor's office this morning, she picked up the telephone and started dialling without asking. She was not able to answer simple questions. The nurses inform you that she is now unable to find her way back to her own room on the ward.

Your consultant is on the phone. He has the results of her MRI scan and wants to discuss the case. In particular, he is interested in:

Your differential diagnosis
Any suggestions you have for further investigations

[advice on page 257]

STATION 11

This 54-year-old butcher attends the A&E department accompanied by his brother. His brother has persuaded him to have his hand looked at as he was punching walls in anger. He believes his wife is having an affair. His brother insists to you in private that she is completely faithful to her husband.

Take a history of delusional jealousy.

[advice on page 260]

STATION 12

You have concerns that a 55-year-old patient has been drinking excessive alcohol over many years. He denies this, but he is happy for you to do a physical examination.

Examine him for the physical stigmata of chronic liver disease.

Tell the patient which physical investigations you would like to do.

[advice on page 263]

STATION 1: BASIC LIFE SUPPORT

THE EXAMINER'S MARK SHEET	
Checking 'ABC'	Background information (if nurse present)
BLS technique	Eyewitness account (if nurse present)
Requesting assistance	Global rating

The patient is unconscious and not breathing.
This is a *medical emergency* and you will score highly if you respond calmly and efficiently. Dithering will not instil the examiner with confidence.

CLINICAL PROCEDURE

Remember to treat a mannequin as if it was a patient.
You will most likely be presented with a 'Resuscitation Annie'.
Based on *Resuscitation Guidelines 2000* (London: Resuscitation Council (UK), 2000).
Remember *ABC:*

1. Ensure safety of the patient and yourself.
2. Check the patient:
    - Does the patient respond?
    - Gently shake shoulder: 'Are you OK?'
3. If the patient does not respond:
    - Shout for help from a nurse
    - Open the *airway*: Gently tilt back the head (care if evidence of neck trauma, e.g. in attempted hanging).
      Remove any visible obstructions from the mouth, e.g. dislodged dentures.
      Lift the chin with your fingertips.
4. Keeping the airway open, look, listen and feel for *breathing*:
    - Look for chest movement, listen for breath sounds.
5. If not breathing:
    - Send someone for help (999, crash team, resus trolley).
    - If on your own, leave the patient for the shortest possible time to get help, return and start rescue breathing.
    - Give *two* slow *rescue breaths*, each of which should make the chest rise and fall:
      Keep the patient's head tilted and chin lifted.
      Pinch the patient's nose closed with finger and thumb of hand on forehead.
      Open the patient's mouth a little.
      Take a deep breath; place your lips around the patient's mouth, ensuring you have a good seal.

Blow steadily for about 2 seconds and watch the patient's chest rise. Maintain head tilt and chin lift, take your mouth away, and watch for the patient's chest to fall.
- Repeat as above.

6. Assess *circulation*:
- Check for carotid pulse: 10 seconds maximum.

7. If no signs of a circulation, start *chest compressions*:
- Do not apply pressure to the lower tip of the sternum or upper abdomen.
- Depress the sternum 4–5 cm during a compression.

8. *Combine rescue breathing and chest compressions*:
- Continue in a ratio of 15 compressions to two effective breaths.

Continue as above until assistance (crash team/ambulance) arrives.

THANK THE NURSE (IF PRESENT)

FOR EXTRA MARKS

Ventilations should take 2 seconds each.

Get as much history from the nursing staff as possible, e.g. is this a drug overdose or suicide attempt?

You could initiate pharmacological treatment, e.g. flumazenil in benzodiazepine overdose.

Explain that you would want to use the resus trolley to get a cardiac tracing and start defibrillation if required.

You need to continue resuscitation until:
- Crash team/ambulance arrives
- Subject shows signs of life
- You are completely exhausted

You want nurses to assist in CPR if possible.

Ideally, you would want to protect yourself by using a reservoir bag and mask for ventilation.

If the patient moves or takes a spontaneous breath, check for circulation and continue if needed. Don't leave for longer than 10 seconds before continuing.

Dilated pupils are an unreliable sign, so continue CPR if present.

Mouth-to-nose ventilation can be used if, for example, mouth obstruction cannot be relieved.

If the cervical spine is damaged, as in a hanging attempt, care must be taken to maintain alignment of the head, neck and chest. Use minimal head tilt when opening the airway.

FURTHER INFORMATION

Resuscitation Council (UK): www.resus.org.uk/siteindx.htm.

STATION 2: EATING DISORDER

THE EXAMINER'S MARK SHEET	
Communication/rapport	Weight-loss methods
Diet history	Thoughts regarding food and weight
Weight history	Global rating

INTRODUCE YOURSELF

'Hello, I'm Dr Smith. It's nice to meet you.'

SET THE SCENE

'I understand you've recently been admitted to the ward.'

ASK FOR PERMISSION

'Could I ask you what led to this admission?'

TAKE A DIETARY AND WEIGHT HISTORY: KEY AREAS

Ask whether it would be alright to ask some questions about her weight in the recent past and now.

Weight

'What is the most you have ever weighed?'
'How tall were you then?'
'When was that?'
'Have you been told your BMI?'
'What was the least you ever weighed in the past year?'
'When was that?'
'How much do you think you ought to weigh?'
'What do you think you see when you look in the mirror?'
'Do you perceive yourself as fat or thin?'
'Do you ever take steps to lose weight?'
Exercise: how much, how often, level of intensity? 'How stressed do you feel if you miss a session?'

Current dietary practices

Ask for specifics about amounts, food groups eaten, preparation time, fluids, restrictions
Hoarding food?
Take a typical 24-hour diet history – all meals, breakfast, etc.
Calorie-counting?
Binge-eating? – frequency, amount, triggers

Purging history
Use of laxatives, stimulants (amphetamines), diet pills
Constipation/diarrhoea
Vomiting? – frequency, how long after meals?

'What has been the effect of this on your physical health?'

ASK WHETHER SHE HAS ANY QUESTIONS

THANK HER

FOR EXTRA MARKS

Family history: obesity, AN/BN, depression, substance misuse
Menstrual history
Use of cigarettes, drugs, alcohol

SUPPORT GROUPS/ADVICE

Eating Disorders Association: www.edauk.com
NHS Direct: www.nhsdirect.nhs.uk
www.youngminds.org.uk

STATION 3: ECG INTERPRETATION

THE EXAMINER'S MARK SHEET	
Communication	Advice to staff
ECG features	Answering other questions
ECG interpretation	Global rating

INTRODUCE YOURSELF

Remain professional when dealing with colleagues.

SET THE SCENE

Take your time to look at the ECG tracing.

FIND OUT WHAT THEY ALREADY KNOW

Enquire about the physical state of the patient. Does he have a cardiac history? Does he currently have chest pain or other symptoms?

ECG INTERPRETATION

'This is a 12-lead ECG of Mr ... [comment on the name, age, date and time taken if present on the tracing to ensure they match the patient described].'
Consider:

Rhythm (?sinus – presence of P waves)
Rate (approximately (number of big squares between complexes)/300)
Axis
QRS complex
QT interval (normal range 0.35–0.43 seconds – one small square = 0.04 seconds, one big square = 0.20 seconds)
ST segment
T waves
Conduction abnormalities
Common arrhythmias

Take your time to look at the tracing before reporting back.

Examples of descriptions

'Looking at the rhythm strip, this shows sinus rhythm with a rate of x beats per minute. The QRS axis appears normal.'
'Looking at the chest and limb leads, the most obvious abnormality is ... '
'The QRS complex is within the normal limit of 120 ms [three small squares].'
'The QT interval appears prolonged at approximately x ms – the usual interval is within 400 ms [two large squares]. I would want to calculate the QTc in this case.'

'My main concerns are that this represents neuroleptic-induced ECG changes.'
'I would want to get advice and an interpretation from a medical specialist
registrar or consultant.'

Course of action if the ECG is abnormal

Many neuroleptic drugs are associated with ECG changes, and some are thought
to increase the cardiac QT interval. This may be a risk factor for torsade de
pointes, a serious ventricular arrhythmia that can be life-threatening.

In the first instance, make sure that the patient is physically well. Is he
complaining of any chest pain or other cardiovascular symptoms? If so, then
potentially this is a medical emergency, and stabilisation and transfer to A&E
should be organised.

Consider reducing or stopping his neuroleptic medication. Seeking urgent advice
from the medical or cardiology team, and their interpretation of the ECG, are
important. You should try to get hold of a previous ECG tracing from his notes
or by contacting previous teams or his GP.

THANK THEM

NOTE

The ECG shown here shows an anterior myocardial infarction. There is ST
elevation in the anterior leads, with Q waves in V1–V3.

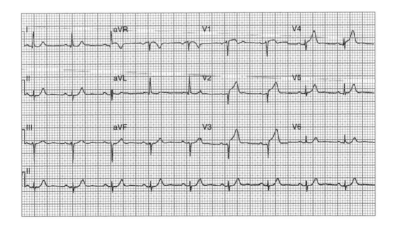

FOR EXTRA MARKS

Potential causes of prolonged QT interval

Drugs: antipsychotics, e.g. pimozide
antidepressants, e.g. amitriptyline
anti-arrhythmics, e.g. amiodarone
others, e.g. erythromycin, chloroquine
Metabolic: hypokalaemia
hypocalcaemia
Others: female
old age
stress

QT interval
The QT interval (usually QTc) is useful but imprecise as a gauge of risk in relation to risk of ventricular arrhythmias and sudden cardiac death (*Drug Saf* 2001; 24: 323–51).
A QTc interval over 500 ms is associated with an increased risk of arrhythmia.
Normal QTc upper limits: men, 440 ms; women, 470 ms.
QTc is calculated using Bazzet's correction formula:

$$QTc = \frac{QT \text{ interval in seconds}}{\sqrt{RR \text{ interval in seconds}}}$$

Drugs can also cause
Heart block
Atrial fibrillation
T-wave changes

FURTHER READING

Hampton JR. *The ECG Made Easy.* Edinburgh: Churchill Livingstone, 2003.

STATION 4: STIMULANT USE

THE EXAMINER'S MARK SHEET	
Communication	Features of dependence syndrome
Empathy	Answering other questions
Appropriate history	Global rating

INTRODUCE YOURSELF

'Hello, I'm Dr Smith. It's nice to meet you.'

SET THE SCENE

'Thank you for coming today.'
'You've reported to us that you have been using stimulants. Is that right?'
'Could we talk about your use of drugs?'

ASK FOR PERMISSION

'Would that be OK?'

TAKE A HISTORY OF STIMULANT USE: KEY AREAS

This is not an obscure OSCE. Due to the rapid rise of crack cocaine use in urban areas, this could well come up. All the same features of dependence apply to stimulants as with alcohol (see Exam 4, Station 3).

Dependence

How long has this man been using stimulants? Is it on a daily basis?
Has his use increased over time?
Stereotyped behaviour?
Compulsion to use stimulants?
Periods of abstinence? Withdrawal phenomena?
Tolerance?
Reinstatement afterwards?
Decline of other activities?

The pattern of stimulant use is usually more spectacular. People can spend months in crack-houses smoking crack continually, presenting to services only at the end, when they are physically exhausted and malnourished.

Ask about route of administration – stimulants can be swallowed, smoked and injected.
Ask about any forms of treatment he has had for his drug-taking.

Consider polysubstance misuse

'Speed-balling' is the co-administration of heroin and cocaine by injection and is common in severe drug-users.

Ecstasy (MDMA)

Amphetamine (speed)

Powdered cocaine, crack cocaine

Risk

Always consider the complications of drug misuse.

ASK WHETHER HE HAS ANY QUESTIONS

THANK HIM

FOR EXTRA MARKS

Don't forget that enquiring about the features of dependence is important for all substances, regardless of whether they are viewed as causing dependence.

FURTHER READING

Kaplan CD, Husch JA, Bieleman B. The prevention of stimulant misuse. *Addiction* 1994; **89**: 1517–21.

STATION 5: KORSAKOFF'S SYNDROME

THE EXAMINER'S MARK SHEET	
Communication	Other features
Empathy	Answering other questions
Memory deficits	Global rating

INTRODUCE YOURSELF

'Hello, I'm Dr Smith. It's nice to meet you.'

SET THE SCENE

'I wanted to talk to you about your memory today.'

ASK FOR PERMISSION

'Would that be OK?'

KORSAKOFF'S SYNDROME: KEY AREAS

You will need to demonstrate the memory difficulties in Korsakoff's syndrome:

Inability to learn and recall new information
Difficulty recalling previously learnt factual knowledge

Immediate recall and procedural memory are preserved.

'How do you think your memory has been lately?'
'Could I test your memory?'
'Some of the things I'm going to ask you will be quite straightforward but others will be difficult, so try not to worry if you make a few mistakes.'

Immediate recall

Digit span (immediate memory): digits are spoken aloud at a rate that allows the patient to memorise them and repeat them back to the examiner. Always start with three digits to assess whether the patient has severe difficulty. Move along to five, six and seven digits.
Classically, the patient can recall digits correctly immediately.

Learning and recalling new information

This is usually tested by giving the patient a name and address to memorise; the patient is asked to recall the name and address immediately and then 5 minutes later. It is likely that the patient will be unable to perform this simple task at 5 minutes. Thus, new learning is severely impaired.

Remote recall

Intermediate memory and memory for relatively remote events (weeks or months) are lost. However, more remote memory sometimes survives.

Ask the patient about some recent current affairs issues to assess the previous weeks. Note the possibility of confabulation. Finally, ask about the past few months.

As a consequence of this amnesia, there is associated disorientation in time.

Other features

Reduced insight: the patient is often unaware or unconcerned by their presentation. Ask whether his memory problems are a concern for him.

Apathy: reduced energy levels and initiative are common-place. Relatives often complain of this before frank memory problems.

Reduced interest in alcohol: often a feature at this stage.

ASK WHETHER HE HAS ANY QUESTIONS

THANK HIM

FOR EXTRA MARKS

Korsakoff first published reports of amnestic disorder in the late 1800s. These cases were the result of thiamine deficiency secondary to persistent high-dose alcohol intake.

Korsakoff's syndrome may be permanent if it follows severe or repeated episodes of encephalopathy.

Wernicke's and Korsakoff's syndromes are likely to be different stages of the same disease process.

Individuals who have severe memory loss can fill gaps unconsciously with false memories (confabulation). Often, they cannot distinguish real memories from those that they have made up. Confabulation is not a prerequisite for a diagnosis of Korsakoff's syndrome.

Korsakoff's syndrome is classified under 'amnesic syndrome' in ICD-10 (F10.6)

FURTHER READING

McIntosh C, Chick J. Alcohol and the nervous system. *J Neurol Neurosurg Psychiatry* 2004; **75** (Suppl 3): 16–21.

STATION 6: ANTIDEPRESSANT TREATMENT

THE EXAMINER'S MARK SHEET	
Communication	Imparting antidepressant information
Empathy	Answering other questions
Reasons prescribed	Global rating

INTRODUCE YOURSELF

'Hello, I'm Dr Smith. It's nice to meet you.'

SET THE SCENE

'Thank you for coming to see me today.'
'Can you tell me why the doctor who saw you suggested you start an antidepressant?'

FIND OUT WHAT HE ALREADY KNOWS

'Can I start by asking you what you already know about antidepressants?'
Has any other professional discussed the pros and cons with the patient?

INFORMATION ON ANTIDEPRESSANTS

Informed choice is an important concept. It is the doctor's responsibility to impart concise, accurate and relevant information for the patient to make the best decision for them as to whether they want to take medication or not. You should do the following:

Talk about the different groups of antidepressants available (in simple lay terms). Discuss the potential benefits and common side effects.
Talk about transient increased anxiety on commencement of SSRIs.
Do not prescribe a 'dangerous' antidepressant when there is a perceived risk of suicide.
Ask whether they have any strong preferences (e.g. is weight gain a concern?).
Discuss the average response times (2–4 weeks), normal course of treatment and likely length of treatment once symptoms resolve (at least 6–12 months after resolution of symptoms).

Current issues with regard to antidepressants that could come up include the following:

Are antidepressants addictive?

This is not a simple question. The answer used to be 'no', but now there are reports that some individuals experience a dependence-like state.

The best answer is: 'People who are on antidepressants for a long time sometimes experience difficulty coming off them, but the majority do not. We would stop any antidepressant gradually, so that hopefully you wouldn't experience withdrawal effects or what we also call discontinuation symptoms.'

Do antidepressants cause suicide?

The best answer is: 'There have been reports of a small minority experiencing increased suicidal ideation with some medications. However, in the vast majority, it has not been a problem.'

(This issue is changing, so keep an eye on the latest findings for the best 'current' response to this question.)

ASK WHETHER HE HAS ANY OTHER QUESTIONS

THANK HIM

FOR EXTRA MARKS

The instructions at this station are deliberately vague, as has occurred in previous examinations. It is important to clarify with the patient their current circumstances, i.e. 'Now, I just wanted to clarify with you: am I correct in saying that you have never taken antidepressant medication before?'

Some patients ask about taking supplements with their medication. Most are OK, but all should be checked out. St John's Wort, for example, is thought to cause both serotonin and noradrenalin re-uptake inhibition, so it should be avoided in order to prevent a serotonin syndrome.

You don't need to know doses or all the names of the medications in the different classes. Just a simple overview – enough to explain in simple terms to a patient – will do. Knowing the common class side effects (the first three or four listed in the *BNF*) is adequate. If you run into trouble, tell the patient: 'I will look into this and get back to you as soon as possible.'

FURTHER READING

Ellis P. Australian and New Zealand clinical practice guidelines for the treatment of depression. *Aust N Z J Psychiatry* 2004; 38: 389–407.

STATION 7: HYPERPROLACTINAEMIA

THE EXAMINER'S MARK SHEET	
Communication	Advice to patient
Empathy	Answering other questions
Explaining hyperprolactinaemia	Global rating

INTRODUCE YOURSELF

'Hello, I'm Dr Smith. It's nice to meet you.'

SET THE SCENE

An empathetic approach is crucial here.
Explain that you understand it is embarrassing and upsetting, but that she has done the right thing by asking to see you.

FIND OUT WHAT SHE ALREADY KNOWS

Ask whether she ever had her blood taken for something called a 'prolactin level'. Were any of the possible side effects of the medication (amisulpride) ever explained to her?
Explain that the amisulpride can sometimes have this side effect and is the most likely cause. Apologise if this was not mentioned to her as a possible side effect when she started the drug.

INFORMATION ON HYPERPROLACTINAEMIA

Explain that: 'Sometimes medication can cause an excess of a naturally produced hormone called prolactin. We usually like to measure prolactin levels in the blood so this doesn't happen. High prolactin levels in the blood are not dangerous but they can have an effect on some of the body's natural processes, like producing breast milk, for example. Some women who have a high prolactin also notice that their periods stop or they lose their sex drive.' (In males, gynaecomastia, and hypogonadism.)
Ask the last time she had a breast examination by a nurse or doctor. Explain that it is very important for her to have her breasts examined and that you will make an urgent appointment for her to see her GP.
If she asks why, explain that anyone who is lactating but is not breastfeeding should have a breast examination to exclude other possible causes, e.g. breast cancer. Make it clear to her that in her case, the medication seems the most likely cause, so she should try not to worry.
Explain that you would also like to take a blood test to measure her prolactin levels.

'If this is the drug, then what do we do next?'

Discuss with the patient and consider her preferences:

If she is prepared to do so, then she could continue on the same drug at a lower dose.

A switch may be necessary if lowering the dose is ineffective.

Switch to a drug with less propensity to elevate prolactin, such as quetiapine or clozapine.

If still not effective, consider adding amantadine or bromocriptine (seek senior input).

Ensure physical causes are excluded.

ASK WHETHER SHE HAS ANY OTHER QUESTIONS

THANK HER

FOR EXTRA MARKS

Risperidone, amisulpride and zotepine increase prolactin significantly.
Prolactin is under the inhibitory control of dopamine.
Hyperprolactinaemia increases osteoporosis risk.
Raised basal prolactin > 390 mU/L.

Medical causes of elevated plasma prolactin

Pituitary disease (prolactinoma)
Chronic renal failure
Hypothyroidism
Sarcoid

Physiological causes of elevated plasma prolactin

Pregnancy
Breastfeeding
Stress
Breast carcinoma can cause galactorrhoea

FURTHER READING

Hummer M, Huber J. Hyperprolactinaemia and antipsychotic therapy in schizophrenia. *Curr Med Res Opin* 2004; **20**: 189–97.

STATION 8: RISK ASSESSMENT

THE EXAMINER'S MARK SHEET	
Communication skills	Risk assessment (self/others)
Empathy	Answering other questions
Self-harm details	Global rating

INTRODUCE YOURSELF

'Hello, my name is Dr. Smith. I'm one of the psychiatrists.'

SET THE SCENE

'Could we talk about what happened yesterday?'
The patient sounds like he wants to leave as soon as possible. He might be dismissive of the seriousness of the attempt on his own life. Gently push him to answer direct questions if he is avoidant.

ASK FOR PERMISSION

'Would that be OK?'

RISK ASSESSMENT: KEY AREAS

Risk to self

As in Exam 1, Station 12, try to determine the details of the overdose:

Where was the overdose taken?
When was the overdose taken?
Who (if anyone) was with them?
What precautions were taken to avoid discovery?

Ask about the ligature marks on his neck and again determine the details.
An attempted hanging is considered very high risk.

Assess the seriousness of the death wish (passive or fully intentional)
Asses his mood, including thoughts and intentions of self-harm
Psychosis: presence of delusional beliefs, command hallucinations or other abnormal perceptions?
Previous self-harm – seriousness
Use of alcohol/drugs
Unemployment
Relationships: single/widowed/divorced/problem
Any supportive relationships?
Compliance with previous interventions, services, etc.

Risk to others

Previous violence: details needed – where, when, whom, prosecuted?

Evidence of rootlessness or 'social restlessness', e.g. few relationships, frequent changes of address or employment?

Use of disinhibiting substances or other potential disinhibiting factors, e.g. social background promoting violence. Note particularly stimulant and crack cocaine use.

Evidence of recent severe stress, particularly of loss events?

Evidence of disengagement from psychiatric aftercare?

Evidence of poor adherence with treatment or of discontinuing medication?

Important mental state issues

Is there evidence of any threat/control-override symptoms, e.g. firmly held beliefs of persecution by others (persecutory delusions), or of mind or body being controlled or interfered with by external forces (delusions of passivity)?

Does the patient have access to potential victims (particularly individuals identified in mental state abnormalities) or to weapons, e.g. guns, swords, knives. Tell-tale signs of deviance include collections of deviant pornography (indicator of sexual threat).

Ask about emotions related to violence, e.g. irritability, anger, hostility, suspiciousness.

Are any specific threats made by the patient?

ASK WHETHER HE HAS ANY QUESTIONS

THANK HIM

FOR EXTRA MARKS

FURTHER READING

Special Working Party on Clinical Assessment and Management of Risk. *Assessment and Clinical Management of Risk of Harm to Other People.* London: Royal College of Psychiatrists, 1996.

STATION 9: RISK ASSESSMENT: SPEAKING TO THE CONSULTANT ON THE PHONE

THE EXAMINER'S MARK SHEET	
Communication	Admit/discharge
Appropriate history	Informal/formal admission
Risk issues	Global rating

INTRODUCE YOURSELF

'Hello, it's Dr Smith here.'

SET THE SCENE

'I've just seen a man in A&E whom I would appreciate discussing with you.'

FIND OUT WHAT THEY ALREADY KNOW

'Do you know anything about him already?'

DISCUSSING RISK ISSUES WITH A COLLEAGUE: REMEMBER TO BE PROFESSIONAL

Consider:

How serious is the risk?
Is the risk specific or general?
Is there an immediate risk?
Best ways to reduce the risk?

Brief history

This will depend on the way that the previous OSCE unfolds. Give the consultant a brief history of the events leading up to this episode of self-harm. Deliver a relevant mental state and risk assessment.

Home situation

The consultant may ask you about the patient's circumstances, e.g. 'If he goes home, who will be there to look after him?'
The seriousness of the attempt would make you reluctant to burden someone with the responsibility for his safety. It would be useful here to know whether the patient describes similar episodes in the past and what happened. The consultant might ask whether you think he could go home with a package of care involving a home-treatment team. Together with someone at home, the case

might be made for discharge. Don't be unduly swayed: they may be pushing you. Remember to always play it safe.

The consultant may then ask you what you would like to do with this patient.

Discuss an admission

Again, this will depend on the previous OSCE. However, an attempted hanging is a serious act of self-harm. Always play safe and, for the purposes of the exam, err on the side of caution. Make the case to the consultant for an admission. Base this on the risk factors that you will have elicited previously, including both a drug overdose and an attempted hanging. In the unlikely event that the consultant refuses an admission, suggest that you might get the specialist registrar to review the case first.

Mental Health Act assessment

The consultant is then likely to ask you whether you think the patient should be admitted formally or informally (in England and Wales, under a section of the Mental Health Act). Having recommended that the patient needs an inpatient assessment, if the patient refuses an informal admission, explain that you believe the risk is such that he should be assessed for detention under the Mental Health Act.

THANK YOUR CONSULTANT

FOR EXTRA MARKS

Be definite and confident (but not arrogant) about the course of action that should be taken.

FURTHER INFORMATION/ADVICE

For information on the Mental Health Act, mental health law and related matters, see www.markwalton.net

STATION 10: NEUROPSYCHIATRIC LUPUS (SLE)

THE EXAMINER'S MARK SHEET	
Communication	Answering other questions
Differential diagnosis	Preferred diagnosis
Investigations	Global rating

INTRODUCE YOURSELF

'Hello, it's Dr Smith here.'

SET THE SCENE

Speak to your consultant on the phone. Explain your concerns as the patient has deteriorated further (this can also buy you a little thinking time!).
'Thank you for calling.'
'This young woman seems to have deteriorated and is now disoriented and inappropriate.'

FIND OUT WHAT THEY ALREADY KNOW

'Have you been updated by the staff?'

INFORMATION ON SLE

This station is meant to test your ability to be logical in the face of a tricky case, rather than your SLE knowledge. Remember: if you are having difficulty, then it is likely that the candidates before and after you will have trouble too. By taking a sensible approach and not panicking you will pass, even if you don't make the diagnosis.

Differential diagnosis

'This case seems to have an organic aetiology. Although failure to respond to two atypical antipsychotics may point towards treatment resistance, the progressive cognitive decline is unlikely to be functional.'
Suggested differential diagnosis in such a case:

Drugs, e.g. steroids
Infection, e.g. HIV, encephalitis
Metabolic disorder
Intracerebral pathology, e.g. space-occupying lesion
Neuropsychiatric
CJD
Schizophrenia

Investigations

Repeat routine testing, plus:

ESR, CRP, thyroid function tests, B12, folate
Infection screen, including HIV, syphilis, hepatitis
Connective tissue screen, including rheumatoid factor and ANA
Neuroimaging (CT/MRI)
EEG
CXR (if not already done)

LIKELY FURTHER INTERACTION WITH THE LATEST CONSULTANT

He tells you that the laboratory has phoned him with blood results showing that the patient is ANA-positive, and an MRI scan shows multiple high-signal white-matter changes affecting both frontal lobes.

What is the diagnosis?
What investigations could you do to confirm this diagnosis?

Diagnosis

Neuropsychiatric lupus (SLE) – a connective tissue disorder.

Further investigations

In addition to the MRI and ANA, lupus is associated with antibodies for double-stranded DNA. Low complement levels suggest active disease and anti-ribosomal P antibody levels have been shown to be useful as a marker of disease activity.

THANK YOUR CONSULTANT

FOR EXTRA MARKS

The neuropsychiatric complications of lupus are rarely the first presenting features of this disease. Commonly, other clinical signs such as skin changes appear first.

Neuropsychiatric symptoms occur commonly in patients with SLE (up to 60 per cent).

Manifestations of CNS involvement in lupus include intractable headaches, generalised seizures, aseptic meningitis, organic brain syndrome, psychosis, severe depression and coma.

The male : female ratio is 1 : 9, and onset usually occurs in early adult life (thirties).

High signal changes on MRI reflect the vasculitic process.

The medical team (rheumatologists) should be informed with regard to treatment and ongoing care.

FURTHER READING

Bodani M, Kopelman MD. A psychiatric perspective on the therapy of psychosis in systemic lupus erythematosus. *Lupus* 2003; 12: 947–9.

STATION 11: DELUSIONAL JEALOUSY

THE EXAMINER'S MARK SHEET	
Communication	Risk issues
Empathy	Answering other questions
History of jealousy	Global rating

INTRODUCE YOURSELF

It is important to state who and what you are, i.e. part of the psychiatric team. He may not want to see a psychiatrist, so this might be a difficult station.

SET THE SCENE

The man is attending A&E for an injured hand, so start with general enquiries, e.g. 'I can see you've hurt your hand.'

ASK FOR PERMISSION

'Can we talk about what happened?'
As sufferers of morbid jealousy can be aggressive, you should mention that you have been asked to see him. Then ask whether he is happy to talk to you. It is very unlikely that the actor will repeatedly say no.

TAKE A HISTORY OF DELUSIONAL JEALOUSY: KEY AREAS

The key feature to demonstrate is an abnormal belief that the partner is being unfaithful on the basis of unsound evidence and reasoning.
It is worth noting that jealousy is common ... as is adultery.

Thoughts and beliefs

A history of progressive and increased preoccupation with infidelity should become evident.
Ask how he knows his wife is being unfaithful.
Does he have any evidence?
Try to assess whether his beliefs are held with delusional intensity.
What does his wife say in response to accusations?
Does he believe her? Why not?

Behaviours

What activities has he been involved in searching for evidence?
Classically, people search through the partner's clothing, including underwear, in an attempt to find 'evidence'.
Often, they will follow their partners without their knowledge (private detective?).

Perceptions

Ask about abnormal perceptions, in particular auditory/command hallucinations.

If present, what do they involve?
'What does the voice tell you to do?'

Risk

Morbid jealousy is associated with violence and murder. You must consider risk and ask him directly whether he plans to harm himself, his wife or anyone else. Someone he believes is involved intimately with his wife might be at considerable risk.
The occupation (butcher) of the man, with access to potential weapons, also suggests danger. Does he have any intention of using knives or implements to harm anyone?

His aggressive outburst leading to a hand injury should be explored.
Is there a past history of morbid jealousy, violence or aggressive acts?
How does he generally get on with his wife (arguments/violence?)?
Have the police ever been involved with domestic problems or violence?
Has he ever confronted his wife?

Sometimes, a partner will falsely admit to having an affair to avoid further accusations or violence. This often makes the situation worse.

Insight

The description suggests that this butcher has very little insight into his current difficulties.
Does he think professional input might be of benefit?

Co-morbidity

Morbid jealousy can occur as an isolated delusional disorder or co-morbidly with a number of other clinical conditions.
If time permits, try to elicit features of schizophrenia, alcohol dependence or paranoid personality disorder.

ASK WHETHER HE HAS ANY QUESTIONS

THANK HIM

FOR EXTRA MARKS

Morbid jealousy is also known as delusional jealousy, pathological jealousy and Othello syndrome.

As in this case, the sufferer is typically middle-aged and the delusionary state is preceded by suspicious preoccupation.

Alcohol abuse tends to shorten the time between diagnosis and violence and prospective crime, such as murder. Therefore, stress the importance of alcohol in the history-taking. Consider performing the CAGE questionnaire.

FURTHER READING

Mullen PE, Martin J. Jealousy: a community study. *Br J Psychiatry* 1994; 14: 35–43.

STATION 12: LIVER DISEASE

THE EXAMINER'S MARK SHEET	
Communication/rapport	Auscultation
Inspection	Investigations
Palpation/percussion	Global rating

INTRODUCE YOURSELF

'Hello, I'm Dr Smith. It's nice to meet you.'

SET THE SCENE

'I have been asked to examine your stomach/tummy.'

ASK FOR PERMISSION

'Would that be OK?'

'If at any point you are uncomfortable or want me to stop, please tell me.'

'I normally have a nurse with me when I examine a patient, but are you happy for me to continue?' (This informs the examiner that ordinarily you would request a chaperone.)

CLINICAL PROCEDURE

Remember: inspection, palpation, percussion and auscultation.

Inform him that you will need to see his chest and abdomen. 'Would that be alright?'

Ask the patient if he can lie flat, arms by his sides.

Expose the abdomen (and chest if male).

Has he had any pain anywhere?

You should perform an abdominal examination (see Exam 2, Station 3), paying particular attention to the following:

Face:	scleral icterus
	telangiectasia
	xanthelasma (prolonged cholestasis)
	cushingoid facies
Hands:	clubbing
	leuconychia (white nails)
	palmer erythema
	Dupuytren's contracture
	hepatic flap (indicating liver cell failure)
Skin:	spider naevi
	loss of axillary hair
	jaundice

Abdomen: hepatomegaly (*a cirrhotic liver may be dull to percussion and small*)
splenomegaly
ascites
Endocrine: gynaecomastia
atrophic testes

Investigations

Explain the reasons for the following investigations:
'I think we should do some blood tests to start with, as I want to see how well your liver is working.'

FBC, including platelet count
LFTs, including GGT
Prothrombin time (clotting)

To exclude other causes of liver failure:

Hepatitis B and C markers
Serum auto-antibodies (lupoid hepatitis, primary biliary cirrhosis)
Serum iron and ferritin (haemochromatosis)
Serum alpha-fetoprotein (malignancy)
Ultrasound liver

Referral to the hepatologists may be indicated if you believe the patient has liver disease.

THANK HIM

FOR EXTRA MARKS

An albumin of < 25 g/L is a poor prognostic factor.
Albumin synthesis is impaired in cirrhosis.
Cirrhosis is a diffuse liver abnormality characterised by fibrosis and abnormal nodular regeneration.
Liver enlargement should be recorded in centimetres below the costal margin, the mid-clavicular line.

INDEX

Note: references are given in the form of the exam number with the station number in brackets. 'vs' indicates the differential diagnosis of two or more conditions.